GUT HEALTH FOR WOMEN

HOW A PLANT-BASED DIET CAN PREVENT
COMMON STOMACH ISSUES, IMPROVE
DIGESTION, DECREASE INFLAMMATION, AND
AID IN WEIGHT LOSS

SHANE CORBITT

© Copyright Shane Corbitt 2021 - All rights reserved.

The content contained within this book may not be reproduced, duplicated or transmitted without direct written permission from the author or the publisher.

Under no circumstances will any blame or legal responsibility be held against the publisher, or author, for any damages, reparation, or monetary loss due to the information contained within this book, either directly or indirectly.

Legal Notice:

This book is copyright protected. It is only for personal use. You cannot amend, distribute, sell, use, quote or paraphrase any part, or the content within this book, without the consent of the author or publisher.

Disclaimer Notice:

Please note the information contained within this document is for educational and entertainment purposes only. All effort has been executed to present accurate, up to date, reliable, complete information. No warranties of any kind are declared or implied. Readers acknowledge that the author is not engaged in the rendering of legal, financial, medical or professional advice. The content within this book has been derived from various sources. Please consult a licensed professional before attempting any techniques outlined in this book.

By reading this document, the reader agrees that under no circumstances is the author responsible for any losses, direct or indirect, that are incurred as a result of the use of the information contained within this document, including, but not limited to, errors, omissions, or inaccuracies.

CONTENTS

FREE PLANT-BASED COOKBOOK

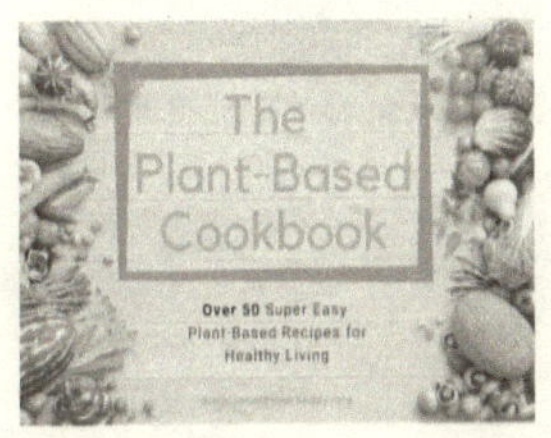

A Free Gift to My Readers

Over 50 Plant-Based Recipes. Download and Start Eating
Healthy Today!

www.createyourhappy.org/cookbook

INTRODUCTION

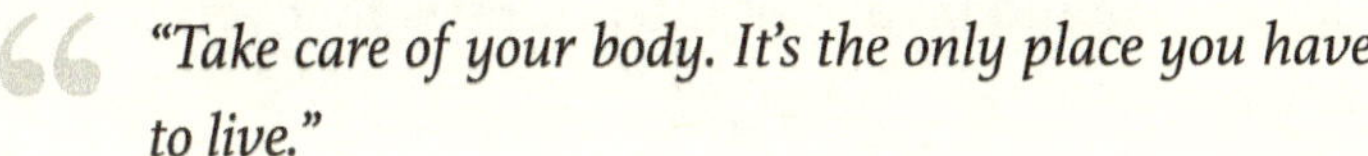

— JIM ROHN

Did you know that more than 100 trillion bacteria reside in your gut? Well, these bacteria play a vital role in your health. Your overall health and metabolism are highly dependent on the microorganisms' activities in your gut. The intestinal bacteria partly consume the dietary fiber you eat as they break them down even further. The breakdown of dietary fiber by the gut bacteria results in the production of inflammatory fatty acids that are required by your body as energy sources. These bacteria are also involved in forming vitamins B and K (Eat the 80, n.d.). Please note that as much as there are beneficial bacteria in your gut, harmful bacteria also exist. You, therefore, need to ensure that your harmful, disease-causing microorganisms are eliminated from your digestive system. Eating probiotics can significantly help with that.

Interestingly, 70% of your immune system operates from your gut (Eat the 80, n.d.). In other words, an overall weak immune system implies that something is not right in your digestive system. As an extension, what you consume directly affects the health of your gut and hence, your immune system's functionalities. As long as there is balance in your digestive system, optimum detoxification, nourishment, and immunity are guaranteed. Your gut is also connected to your brain to such an extent that it can affect your mood and behaviors. Having said this, taking good care of your gut should be one of the priorities that you uphold with dignity.

Why Plant-Based Diets?

Plant-based diets, including vegan and fruitarian ones, have gained momentum over the years. Even celebrities like Jay Z, Venus Williams, Bill Clinton, Beyonce, and Liam Hemsworth have adopted this diet as part of their lifestyles. There are various reasons why plant-based diets are increasingly becoming more preferred than other eating patterns, and we will explore some of them in this section.

- **Caring for animal welfare:** Animals are often exploited for food and other purposes by human beings. Plant-based diets are an alternative to meat, so they help preserve animals. Activists for animals suggest that animals also have a right to live just like humans do. Therefore, instead of depending on animals for food, humans can look elsewhere, that is, to plants.

- **The numerous health benefits:** Eating a diet that is predominantly plant-based reduces the chances of conditions like high cholesterol levels, type 2 diabetes, high blood pressure, and some cancers. Consuming meat exposes your body to higher concentrations of nitrates that may trigger the initiation of some cancers. Fruits, grains, and vegetables contain phytocompounds like beta-carotene, enhancing eye vision. Some of the compounds in plants reduce inflammation and strengthen your bones.

- **Affordability:** It is undeniably true that meat and other animal products are pretty expensive compared to plant foods. The cost of red meat, pork, and chicken is far higher than fruits, grains, and vegetables. This means that you are more likely to save some dollars, rands, euros, or whichever currency if you replace the meat in your diet with plant-based foods. Nuts, legumes, quinoa, seeds, and dark leafy vegetables will still provide you with the proteins you look for in meat but at a much lower cost. Would you imagine that a $0.99 meal of lentils would feed four people? That is unlikely to happen with animal-based products.

We Got You Covered!

Gut issues can be frustrating, especially considering the irritation that they come with. I understand why you are so desperate to correct the discrepancies in the functionality of your gut as soon as possible. Whether as a short-term disease or chronic illness, gut-related problems are not something to condone. The proper plant-based diet is probably all you need to deal with gut illnesses once and for all. Sounds great, right? Yes, but here is another challenge that you might be facing. Do you know how to transition yourself to start eating a plant-based diet from the eating patterns that you have been following all along? Maybe not, but not to worry. This book will provide you with a complete guide that helps you smoothly and gradually change your diet to a plant-based one.

Perhaps you are not sure whether your gut is OK or not. This book will begin by enlightening you on the components of the gut that you should know. This will form a proper foundation for understanding how your gut functions. Enlightenment on the proper functionalities of your gut will assist you to quickly notice should there be any abnormalities in the way your digestive system should work. Like they say, "Knowledge is power." This book will empower you to make informed decisions about your health, particularly your gut health.

While some sources have presented a plant-based diet as something that needs perseverance, here we introduce this diet as part of a healthy lifestyle.

Meet the Author

Shane Corbitt is an expert in nutrition and weight loss who has authored the book with the title *A Beginner's Guide to Sustainable Plant-Based Weight Loss*. Having had his own share of personal struggles with eating the right foods for his health. Shane developed a burden to share the right information with regard to healthy and sustainable eating patterns and styles. Shane loves to help women break free from diets that are not very supportive of their good health. Shane also desires to see women reach their long-awaiting goals without having to struggle with fad diets or sacrificing their health. He has an unquenchable passion for helping women lead healthy lifestyles for themselves and their families.

Shane is knowledgeable in the subject area that is presented in this book because he has been studying nutrition and weight loss in women for many years. As an extension of his theoretical knowledge, Shane has also worked with many women, guiding them in nutritional aspects. In writing this book, Shane understands diet culture, its benefits, and its struggles. Therefore, he is fully empowered to help women across the globe attain a healthier lifestyle the right way.

1

———

A LOOK INTO THE GUT

While all body parts are important, the gut might be one of the things that you should give extra attention to if you want to maintain a healthy body. You cannot properly break down your food when your digestive system is not healthy. Such a scenario is disastrous because your body would be deprived of the nutrients and energy that it requires to function well. Metabolism is compromised when your body is unable to deal with the food that you eat in an appropriate manner. For you to perfectly understand the importance and role of the gut, let's dive into exactly what the gut is so that you can get familiar with what we are fighting for.

The Gut Through the Ages

The gut is also referred to as the gastrointestinal tract or digestive system. Due to its importance, this system should be protected from changes that come with aging. This is because even in older individuals, breakdown of food, absorption of nutrients, and elimination of waste still need to take place efficiently. However, it has been noted that as time progresses, the digestive tract is characterized by slower functioning and increased vulnerability to gut-related disorders.

One study reported that your digestive system is unlikely to be affected by aging processes up until you reach about 65 years of life (Mayfair, 2019). Let's have a look at the various changes that you might expect as you approach your senior years.

In the Mouth

The salivary glands begin to produce low amounts of saliva. This, accompanied by weaker jaw muscles, will make it more difficult for you to chew food and ultimately swallow it. Chewing is a very crucial part of the whole process of digestion. It helps reduce the size of the food particles for two main reasons. First, to make swallowing the food easier. Second, absorption of nutrients is easier and faster when the food particles are in much smaller sizes. Therefore, the changes that take place in the mouth as you age significantly affect digestion and absorption processes.

In the Esophagus

Soon after the mouth, there is a part called the esophagus, which immediately receives the food that you swallow. The primary role of this part is to channel the food from the mouth to the stomach. Normally, the esophagus has upper and lower esophageal sphincters that open and close to enhance the movement of food from your mouth down to the stomach. The upper esophageal sphincter senses when there is food coming from the mouth, so it opens to let it into the esophagus. The food is then pushed by muscular contractions of the esophagus toward the lower esophageal sphincter, which also opens to release its contents into your stomach. Unfortunately, as years go by, your sphincters, especially the upper one, weaken, and so do the esophageal contractions.

In the Stomach

The stomach is more than just a hollow organ that holds the food that you eat before it's transferred to the intestines. This is where the food is mixed with enzymes that catalyze the further breakdown into even smaller particles. This is a strategy for aiding the efficient absorption of nutrients when the food gets to the intestines. The cells that make up the stomach lining are responsible for the production of the relevant enzymes, along with a strong acid that keeps the environment unconducive to the proliferation of pathogenic microorganisms. It is also important to note that the lining of the stomach is elastic, a property that gives this organ flexibility with regard to how much food it can contain.

In older individuals, the elasticity of the stomach lining might reduce significantly. As a result, it becomes more prone to damage and the development of ulcers. Moreover, the stomach won't be able to accommodate more food when its elasticity is compromised. This means that no matter how much food your body needs, there is only so much that you can eat at any given time, depending on the capacity of your stomach.

In the Small Intestines

The small intestine is a muscular tube that is 22 feet long. It can be divided into three parts: the duodenum, jejunum, and ileum. Further breakdown of the food received from the stomach occurs in the duodenum. Here, the food is mixed together with digestive juices that contain enzymes from the liver and pancreas. The jejunum and ileum are the lower part of the small intestine, and this is where most of the absorption takes place.

The movement of food throughout the small intestine is aided by peristalsis, which is the muscular contractions, similar to what happens in the esophagus. The food enters the small intestines in a semi-solid form but ends up being liquid as it mixes with water, enzymes, bile, and mucus. Aging reduces the levels of lactase in the small intestines. This triggers intolerance of dairy products as time progresses. The absorption of some nutrients, like calcium, vitamin B12, and iron, is affected by the ratios of the microbial flora in the small intestines. Therefore, the increased growth of some bacteria tends to reduce the efficient absorption of such essential nutrients in the body.

In the Large Intestines

The large intestine, also known as the colon, is a muscular tube that stretches as an extension of the small intestines, connecting to the rectum. This tube is about six feet long, and this is where water is absorbed, and waste is processed.

The food from the small intestines enters the large intestines in a liquid form and ends up being solid as water is progressively absorbed. It takes approximately 36 hours for food waste to pass through the large intestine with the aid of peristalsis (Cleveland Clinic, n.d.).

As you age, the movement of contents in the colon becomes relatively slower. This means that it will take longer for you to release waste after eating your food. This can lead to irritation and uncomfortable feelings. You might even experience abdominal pains and reduced appetite.

In the Rectum

Your large intestines empty their contents into the rectum for excretion. The rectum is a chamber that is eight inches in size, and it is the one that is connected to the anus through a sphincter muscle. The primary role of the rectum in the digestive system is to hold the waste that needs to be evacuated until it has been excreted. Once it receives waste from the colon, it lets the body know that there are contents that need to be excreted but until then, it keeps the waste.

For the stool to be released, the sphincter muscle connecting the rectum to the anus should relax while the rectum contracts to push its contents out. The sphincter contracts when you are not ready to release, and the rectum relaxes. As you age, the rectum tends to enlarge. This makes it difficult for the rectum to contract and release the waste when it's full. As a result, aging is usually coupled with increased instances of constipation.

The Location and Structure of the Gut

In the previous section, we have already tapped into some of the nitty-gritty of where the gut is found in the body. This section will give you a brief explanation that enables you to visualize the location of your digestive system in a much simpler sense.

Generally, your gastrointestinal tract stretches from your mouth to your anus. In other words, you consume your food through the mouth, and after it has been processed, it is excreted through the anus. Here is an outline of the main parts that make up your digestive system:

- **Mouth:** Your teeth, saliva, and salivary enzymes are the main components that aid digestion in the mouth. The main enzyme active in the mouth is salivary amylase, which is responsible for breaking down starch. Saliva helps to mix the food with the enzymes that are available in the mouth.
- **Gullet:** This is the esophagus. This part is located in your neck region. The walls of this muscular tube contract each time you swallow food.
- **Stomach:** This is the third part of the digestive system. It marks the connection between the gullet and the small intestines.
- **Small intestines:** The duodenum is the upper part of the small intestines, connected to the stomach. It is then followed by the jejunum and then the ileum. The duodenum literally continues with the function of the stomach as it further breaks down the food

that you ate. This part of the small intestines can be identified as a c-shaped tube that is coiled around the pancreas. The jejunum and the ileum are also coiled at the center of your abdomen.

- **Large intestines:** This is the last part of the gastrointestinal tract and is made up of the ascending colon, transverse colon, descending colon, and rectum. The sole function of the large intestine is to absorb water and get rid of waste.

The Role of the Gut

The gut processes food so that it is either absorbed or excreted. In a nutshell, the main functions of the digestive tract are digestion, absorption, and excretion. We will discuss these functions further in this section.

Digestion

Digestion refers to the breakdown of food particles into smaller ones that are easier to manage. The gut facilitates two types of digestion. These are

- **Mechanical digestion:** Mechanical digestion describes the processes during which the digestive system physically aids the breakdown of food particles. Chewing food in the mouth is an excellent example of mechanical digestion. The same applies to food churning that takes place in the stomach, as well as segmentation in the small intestines. Peristalsis in the esophagus and the small and large intestines are also part of mechanical digestion.

Mechanical digestion helps to release nutrients that are trapped within food particles.

- **Chemical digestion:** Chemical digestion is the breakdown of food particles that is catalyzed by digestive enzymes. Nutrient molecules are held together by chemical bonds. Digestive enzymes are capable of breaking these bonds, thereby releasing nutrients in forms that the body is able to use. For example, proteins are broken down into amino acids, and complex carbohydrates are reduced into simpler sugars.

Absorption

Unless nutrients are absorbed into the bloodstream for use, then the digestion process is irrelevant. So, when both mechanical and chemical digestion has taken place, carbohydrates, fats, proteins, vitamins, and minerals are absorbed into the bloodstream before they are distributed to parts of the body where they will be used.

Excretion

When nutrients and water have been absorbed by the body, the remaining residue is excreted. It is the role of your gastrointestinal tract to eliminate waste and create space for more food. The excretion process by the gut is so efficient to the extent that only materials that your body will no longer need or those that will be toxic to you if they stay longer are eliminated.

Contributes to the Immune System

The microorganisms that reside in the gut, also known as the gut microbiota, help regulate a balance in the immune system. Recent studies have confirmed that the bacteria in the gut play crucial roles in both adaptive and innate immunity (Zheng et al., 2020). Adaptive immunity is described as the protection you have in response to a specific pathogen presented to your body. On the other hand, innate immunity is inborn, nonspecific, and active against all types of invaders in your body.

The gut microbiota trains and also enhances the development of major components of the immune system. In one study that was done by Kathryn Winglee, who is a co-director at the Johns Hopkins Center for Tuberculosis Research Laboratory, revealed that the progression of tuberculosis was associated with changes in bacterial communities in the gut (Fields, 2014). This shows that there is a link between the type and number of microorganisms in your gut and the strength of your immune system.

There are various factors that influence the microbial communities in the gut. These include the type of nutrition, your mother's diet during pregnancy, use of antibiotics, infections, and genetics. An imbalance in types and numbers of microorganisms in the gut, especially in infants, will affect overall health for a lifetime. Some cases of asthma, obesity, allergies, and metabolic disorders are attributed to imbalances in the gut microbiota (Danone Nutricia Research, n.d.).

Contributes to Mood Regulation

Your gut is highly involved in regulating your mood. This is partly explained by the fact that there are approximately 100 million neurons that are found in your gastrointestinal tract (Danone Nutricia Research, n.d.). These neurons release neurotransmitters that are involved in regulating mood and satiety-related aspects. Neurotransmitters are chemical substances that carry messages from one nerve cell to another.

Details of What Happens in Your Gut

Now you have a general understanding of what happens in your gut. We have explained the facts that your gastrointestinal tract is where digestion, absorption, and excretion take place. This section will devolve into further detail regarding the processes that take place in different parts of your gut.

Mouth

Both mechanical and chemical digestion begins in the mouth. Once you eat your food, the first goal is to reduce the food particles into smaller ones that are easier to manage. This is a mechanical process that is aided by your teeth. The more you chew the food, the more it is broken down and mixed with saliva. Your saliva contains enzymes that kick-start the chemical digestion of food in the mouth. One of the enzymes available in your saliva is the salivary amylase, whose role is to break down complex carbohydrates, known as polysaccharides, into simple sugars that your body can use. Your saliva also contains lingual lipase, which is an enzyme that reduces triglycerides to simpler fats. The more the food is mixed with the saliva, the more it is exposed to the salivary enzymes. This also marks the beginning of an efficient digestion process.

Gullet

In the esophagus, mechanical digestion may take place. The contractions of the walls of the gullet as it pushes food toward the stomach further break it down. Otherwise, there isn't any chemical digestion that happens in the gullet.

Stomach

From the time a child is born, the first few years of their existence are coupled by significant changes in the structure and size of the stomach. Can you imagine that a baby's stomach at birth is capable of holding only between five and seven milliliters of milk? Within two or three days, that same stomach would be able to contain about 22 to 27 milliliters of milk, implying an almost four-fold increase in size! By the time a child becomes one month old, their stomach is big enough to hold around 80 to 150 milliliters of milk (Danone Nutricia Research, n.d.). It takes just 30 days for the stomach to achieve a greater than ten-fold increase in volume after birth!

The digestion that takes place in the stomach is predominantly chemical. The cells that line this organ secrete different types of enzymes that act on different components of the food. One of such enzymes that are produced by the cells in the stomach lining is pepsin, whose role is to break down proteins. Gastric lipase is also secreted, targeting the triglycerides in your food. The stomach muscles periodically contract, thereby churning food and enhancing more efficient digestion.

Intestines

Further chemical digestion takes place in the duodenum, which is the upper part of the small intestine. The enzymes that are available in the small intestines are released by the pancreas. Some of the enzymes that are found in the small intestine are sucrase, the enzyme that chemically digests sucrose and lactase, which break down lactose (Nall, 2018). In the jejunum and ileum, carbohydrates, proteins, fats, minerals, and vitamins are absorbed into the bloodstream and presented to the body in forms that it can use.

There are no enzymes that are released in the large intestine. The breakdown of nutrients in this part of the gut is aided by the action of the microorganisms that stay there. The absorption of water, minerals, and vitamins takes place in the large intestine.

You see, the gut is not just one part of the body but a connection of different important aspects from the mouth to the intestines. The gut incorporates so many rules, processes, and roles that keep you healthy overall. At this point, you might have had a bunch of biology terms thrown at you to the extent that your brain is probably going into a hyperdrive! Let's give ourselves a break with the next chapter as we talk about some of the most bizarre and interesting facts about our guts.

2

___

THE BIG GUT FACTS

When your gut is working well, it can really do wondrous things that can boggle your mind. Sometimes, we don't really pay attention to our guts and what it can do, but we will notice it when something goes wrong. Your gut will always play a key role in your health, so it's good to know more about it, right? In this chapter, you will gain more insight into various aspects of your gut, both the amazing and the weird.

Fact Number 1: Your Stomach Acid Is So Strong, It Can Burn Your Skin

The acid found in your stomach is called hydrochloric acid, and it is one of the most dangerous acids that can even tear your denim if it comes into contact with it. Not only that, it can even dissolve a metal!

The more surprising part is how such a strong acid can stay in your stomach without burning it. The inner part of your stomach is lined with a protective mucus that shields it from the possible damage by the stomach acid. No other part of your body can tolerate the corrosive effect of hydrochloric acid. Even when inhaled, hydrochloric acid can cause effects such as damage to lung tissue, accumulation of fluid in your lungs, and issues in the upper respiratory tract.

The pH of stomach acid ranges from 1.5 to 3.5 (MedlinePlus, 2013). This low pH confirms the strength of the acid. This acid sometimes leaks back into the gullet, which unfortunately doesn't have the protective mucus layer. This happens when the lower esophageal sphincter is loose or weakened. Such leakages explain what is known as heartburn or acid reflux, where you feel a burning sensation close to your throat area. You might even experience a sour taste in your mouth if the acid reflux is severe.

Fact Number 2: Your Intestines Harbor Detergents

Bile is a digestive liquid that is produced by your liver. This digestive liquid contains bile acids, which aid in the digestion and absorption of fats. Bile acids are the detergents in the intestines. Imagine how fats are difficult to deal with without soap. Also, imagine yourself washing a plate without a detergent. That plate is not going to be clean! So bile acids make it easy for your gut to handle fats.

Without detergent, fats cannot mix with water. By assuming the role of a detergent, bile acids make it possible for fats to mix with water in the gut. It is only then that digestive enzymes can then act upon the fats to break them down into forms that the body can metabolize.

Here is a more interesting comparison between bile acids and common detergents. At a molecular level, all soaps and detergents are amphipathic, which means they have hydrophilic and hydrophobic ends. The hydrophilic end is the one that interacts with water, while the hydrophobic part interacts with fats or dirt. This structure helps the detergent to cause the dirt to mix with the water so that it is rinsed off. Bile acids also have a similar molecular structure. They contain hydrophobic ends, which are lipid-soluble, and hydrophilic ends, which are water-soluble.

Fact Number 3: Prebiotics Can Really Help You

Incorporating prebiotics in your diet is an excellent way of keeping the right microbiota in amounts that maintain the good health of your gut. Prebiotics are food ingredients that are non-digestible and capable of triggering the growth and activity of selected microorganisms in the gastrointestinal tract. This, apart from enhancing the gut's health, also promotes the overall well-being of an individual.

Fiber, being indigestible, is a good and easily-accessible prebiotic. Some studies reported that an increase in fiber intake for about two weeks significantly alters the microbial communities in the gut in a positive way (Huzar, 2021). The bacteria in your gut can act upon the fiber to release chemicals that nourish your body. A diet that is rich in fiber also comes in handy in reducing the probability of having colon cancer. Another study also reported that dietary fiber plays a crucial role in reducing colorectal cancer (Masrul and Nindrea, 2019). There are different mechanisms through which dietary fiber achieves this. These include binding to and diluting fecal carcinogens and increasing the bulkiness of the stool that you excrete. Dietary fiber, as a prebiotic, also reduces the transit time for your stool. This helps to lower the chances of the carcinogens getting into direct contact with the colorectal lining.

Another interesting fact is that short-chain fatty acids are produced when bacteria ferment the fiber that you eat. It is suggested that these fatty acids are capable of protecting you against cancers that affect the gut, particularly colorectal cancer (Masrul and Nindream 2019). Fiber also slows down the absorption of glucose into your bloodstream. This lowers the risk of suffering from diabetes and some types of cancers.

Fact Number 4: Your Gut Microbiota Weighs up to Six Pounds

The bacteria that stays in your intestines, known as the gut microbiota, can weigh up to six pounds. Amazing, right? These bacterial populations can go up to tens of trillions in numbers. However, it is important to note that bacterial communities are not identical in all people.

Before birth, your gut is sterile, but microorganisms develop with time. A remarkable part of the microbial communities in your gut is acquired at infancy as you move down the birth canal in the event of a normal delivery. Therefore, there should be a difference in the gut microbiota of an individual who was born through normal delivery and another delivered through a Caesarian section. The types of antibiotics that you use also impact the types and numbers of bacteria in your intestines, and so does the type of diet that you follow. Do you now see why your gut microbiota is different from that of the person next to you?

Fact Number 5: Gut Microorganisms Can Contribute to Your Emotions and Behavior

The types and numbers of bacteria in your gut might play a role in the emotions you experience and the behaviors you display. *Lactobacillus rhamnosus* is one of such microorganisms, as revealed by some studies. One research endeavor investigated the behavior of mice that were fed with *L. rhamnosus* to determine the possible effects of the microorganisms. From the behavior that the mice exhibited after feeding on *L. rhamnosus*, the researchers deduced that the microorganism altered the brain chemistry of the mice. If *L. rhamnosus* could affect the brain's functioning, how many other bacteria in the gut can?

The American Psychology Association also reported that the bacteria in your gastrointestinal tract are able to release hundreds of neurochemicals (Carpenter, 2021). Your brain detects these neurochemicals and uses them to control some physiological processes in your body. The neurochemicals are also used to regulate mental processes like mood and learning.

The gut microbiota is linked to the regions of the brain that deal with emotions. Plant-based diets are a great way to keep the gut-brain connection healthy. More grains, vegetables, and fruits in your diet will assist the microorganisms in your gut to grow and produce neurochemicals as they should.

Fact Number 6: Your Gut Can Work Without Permission From Your Brain

To a larger extent, your digestive system can act without being triggered by the brain. This is a unique feature of this organ, considering that all the other organs of your body operate in response to impulses from the brain. All the crucial responsibility of digestion is fulfilled by the gut without much input from the brain. For this reason, the gastrointestinal tract can be referred to as an organ that "acts as its own brain" (Rosenfeld, 2018).

How is it that your gut thinks for itself? This is because the walls of your gut contain what we call the "brain in the gut," which scientists call the enteric nervous system (ENS). The ENS can't balance your checkbook or recall a story like what the main brain in your head would do. Its primary role is to regulate the whole process of digestion from the moment you put food in your mouth. The secretion of enzymes that carry out the chemical digestion of your food is controlled by the ENS. This system also regulates the rate at which the blood flows as a way of controlling the absorption of various nutrients into the bloodstream (Johns Hopkins Medicine, 2019). It also regulates the elimination of the waste products of digestion. The gastrointestinal tract contains millions of neurons in its walls throughout its nine-meter stretch. Even the peripheral nervous system or spinal cord does not harbor such large numbers of neurons.

Although the ENS cannot think, it does communicate with the bigger brain to produce results that are beneficial to your overall health. This happens through the vagus nerve, which is a big visceral nerve that is found in your digestive tract. Science reports that about 90% of the vagus nerve fibers carry information from the gastrointestinal tract to the brain. Please note the direction of information movement between the gut and the brain — it's not the other way round. The brain interprets this information that is communicated by the gut through the vagus nerve as emotions.

Fact Number 7: 95% of Your Body's Serotonin is in the Gut

About 95% of the serotonin that your body uses is made by the bacteria that reside in your gut (Carpenter, 2021). Serotonin regulates your happiness, anxiety, and mood, which is why people who suffer from depression and stress have significantly lower amounts of serotonin. In fact, serotonin has antidepressant effects. Other antidepressants that you take in a bid to address low mood and stress are made in resemblance to this molecule. It is, therefore, interesting that you have a greater part of this antidepressant being made in your gut.

One study showed that serotonin is highly involved in communication processes that take place between the brain and gastrointestinal tract. This hormone also helps regulate the rate at which food moves along your digestive system. It also plays a vital role in determining the amount of fluid that is produced in the intestines. This includes mucus, among other fluids that aid digestion and absorption. Serotonin also affects the sensitivity of your intestines to satiation and pain (Case-Lo, 2020).

Fact Number 8: A Healthy Gut Enhances Bone Protection

Some studies in mice revealed that reduced serotonin production is associated with a slowdown in the reduction of bone density that is osteoporosis-related (Stoller-Conrad, 2015). This study marked a foundation for the possible development of new drugs for fighting osteoporosis.

Serotonin has positive effects on bone mass only when the brain produces it. In this case, the neurotransmitter promotes the formation of bones while reducing bone resorption. However, the case is different when the serotonin is secreted in another organ that is outside the brain, the gut included. In this scenario, the production of large amounts of serotonin negatively impacts bone formation (Ducy and Karsenty, 2010). The gut-derived serotonin does this by halting the proliferation of osteoblasts, which are the cells that secrete the substance that bones are made of (Lavoie et al. 2017)

Fact Number 9: The Gut Can Cure Your Cold

Your gut harbors approximately 70% of your immune cells. These immune cells exist as gut-associated lymphoid tissue (GALT), which acts by expelling or destroying pathogenic microorganisms that attack your gut. Therefore, the GALT collaborates with the gut microbiota to protect you from ailments like flu and colds. From this information, you can detect why using antibiotics regularly is not always such a great idea. Antibiotics can kill both the pathogenic and beneficial bacteria in your gut, thereby making you more susceptible to illnesses (Rosenfeld, 2018).

Generally, the immune system is made in such a way that it can identify and recognize viruses that attack your body prior to taking necessary action to destroy them. Your immune system releases chemicals that activate cells that are able to fight against viruses. This also applies to the viruses that cause flu and colds. Now that the bulk of your immune cells is in the gut, this explains the undeniable involvement of the gut in protecting you against the common cold and flu.

A well-balanced gut microbiota does not always mean that you will never catch a cold at all. However, your probability of getting the cold is remarkably reduced. In the event that you catch a cold, the symptoms will be less severe and may not even last long.

Fact Number 10: The Gut Uses the Brain More Than What Speech Does

Your brain has what is called gray matter, which is responsible for processing all the information that is sent to this organ. Some structures are positioned within the gray matter that receive and process signals from different stimuli. The processed information is then sent to the central nervous system, where a response to the original stimuli is triggered. This response could be any appropriate behavior.

Now, did you know that your gut uses the gray matter of your brain more than other functions of the body, such as speech? This shows that a lot of information is communicated to the brain by the gut, which requires processing. Such vast communication also reflects the importance of the gut in your survival as a human being.

Fact Number 11: Your Gut can Diagnose Problems

Tummy rumbles have become the basis for the non-invasive diagnosis of some health issues like Irritable Bowel Syndrome (IBS). This condition affects between 10 to 20% of people, whether male or females, in the United Kingdom (UK) (BBC Radio 4, 2018). In North America, the prevalence of IBS ranges from 3 to 20% (Saito et al., 2002). Even with such prevalence, diagnosing IBS can be quite challenging and invasive.

The gut could be the easiest, cheapest, and more accurate way to determine if you are sick with IBS. This was shown by the Noisy Guts Project that was done in Australia. Through this project, an acoustic belt has been developed, which is capable of recording the noises or rumbles in the gut for a given period of time. These gut noises are then interpreted using computers and algorithms to diagnose the presence of IBS. This method of diagnosis had an 85% success rate as of 2018 (BBC Radio 4, 2018).

Yes, the gut is a marvelous and fascinating thing. There are so many interesting things to learn about the connection of processes that take place within the gut. Learning more about the gut and its health can really help you get into the mindset of what you are fighting for. In the next chapter, we will explore the link between the diet and the gut.

3

THE DIET AND THE GUT

The gut is home to trillions of microorganisms that will help it function properly and efficiently. A healthy diet also helps keep the gut microbiota at stable levels. In this chapter, you will learn the main links that a plant-based diet has with your gut. This will assist you in fully understanding the importance of a nutritious diet. You will also be enlightened on the association between an unhealthy diet and the gut. This chapter will unleash some tips and tricks for keeping your gut healthy with the right food. You will also learn the signs to look out for if things get wrong in your gastrointestinal tract.

The Dietary Influence

For every individual, the unique composition of the microorganisms that reside in the gut is relatively stable. However, some lifestyle factors impact changes in this composition on a daily basis. One of such lifestyle aspects is the type of food that makes up your diet. Research has shown that approximately 50% of the structural changes to gut microbiota are attributed to dietary alterations (Leeming et al., 2019). This also means that changes in your diet affect your gut microbiota. This means that whatever you eat has an influence on the composition of microorganisms in your gastrointestinal tract.

Effects of Dietary Changes on the Gut Microbiota

The gut microbiota can even double every hour, depending on what you eat. Please note that the shifts in the composition of the gut microbiota as a result of dietary changes tend to be temporary. However, this does not mean you should take the changes lightly. The effects of the changes in numbers and composition of the microbial communities in your gastrointestinal tract can be devastating in those short periods of time during which they happen. Sometimes, the changes are quite beneficial to your health and the general functioning of your whole body.

The type of diet you follow determines the kind of nutrients available for the growth and multiplication of the taxa that exists in your gut. Some nutritional compositions will undoubtedly favor the growth of certain microorganisms over others. Your diet also influences the levels of auto-antibodies that are made by your body in preparation for attacks by pathogenic bacteria. Do you see how important your diet is to your health and overall well-being?

Anything that disrupts your eating patterns is more likely to affect your nutritional availability, thereby also affecting your gut's microbial composition. For example, the Circadian cycle of sleep and awakeness can affect your eating patterns. Suppose you are failing to sleep well due to health issues; you might then start to eat food during the time when you would normally be sleeping. This alters the state of microbial communities in your digestive system. Likewise, some research has shown that shift workers who have no choice but to break normal sleeping patterns sometimes experience significant changes in the composition of their gut microbiota (Leeming et al., 2019).

The main factors of your diet that tend to affect your gut microbiota include the time at which you eat and the frequency and duration of the consumption period. These will affect not only the composition of your gut's microbial flora but also its functions. For instance, a study done by a group of researchers showed that food consumption that is done rhythmically leads to a 15% alteration in the composition of commensal bacteria within a 24-hour period (Thaiss et al., 2014). Commensal bacteria are different strains that have a neutral relationship, with no harm involved toward each other. Significant increases in microbial abundance, in general, were also observed in the study that Christoph Thaiss and colleagues did. Simply put, when you take regular meals at the same time every day, your gut microbiota increases in numbers. This also increases their efficiency in their various functions that enhance your well-being.

Do Short-Term Changes in Diet Impact the Gut Microbiota?

Nowadays, people try different dietary patterns for various reasons, including weight-loss endeavors. You can probably relate to such scenarios. As you explore these different dietary exploits, it is essential to note that your gut microflora's composition and functioning abilities are also affected, either positively or negatively. Studies that were done to investigate the effects of short-term changes in diet revealed that not all microorganisms in your gut are affected. Instead, the alterations are limited to some bacterial strains (Thaiss et al., 2014). The rest of the bacterial communities remain the same no matter the changes in the diet.

When you make abrupt changes to your diet, rapid alterations take place in the composition of your gut microbiota, especially within the first 24 hours after the dietary intervention has been implemented. One research was done to investigate the effects of dietary interventions on gut microbiota (David et al., 2014). The participants in the study were subjected to either a plant-based or animal-based diet. The results from the study showed that both diets caused significant changes in the microbial composition of the gut. The animal-based diet was associated with a significant reduction in carbohydrate fermentation and an increase in amino acid fermentation. The opposite was true with the plant-based diet. These changes took place within a 24-hour period. Such results show that animal-based dietary interventions tend to reduce the microbial populations involved in processing carbohydrates. Another interesting finding from the same study was that the microbial state of the participants returned to normal after about three days of the dietary intervention.

The gut microbiota is also altered by changes in levels of macronutrients, as well as other food components. The macronutrients whose effects on the gut microflora are significant are fats, carbohydrates, and proteins. As we mentioned earlier, the fiber content in your diet also impacts the gut's microbial composition. A review that was done in 2018 also supported this notion, confirming that dietary interventions for fiber, like fructans, played a crucial role in increasing the numbers of bacteria such as *Lactobacillus* and *Bifidobacterium* species (So et al., 2018).

The Gut and an Unhealthy Diet

An unhealthy diet affects your well-being. It has components that are not supportive of your physical, mental, and emotional health. Sometimes, a diet becomes unhealthy when it has too high a concentrations of components that would have been non-toxic if they were consumed in their correct proportions. An unhealthy diet poses a threat to the composition of the microorganisms in your gut. This section will start by exploring what an unhealthy diet might include. This will help to clear any misunderstandings with regard to what is and is not unhealthy. We will further enlighten you on what you should look out for to determine if your gut is unhealthy. Not only that, but we will also give you tips on what you can do so that your gastrointestinal tract will become and stay healthy.

Characteristics of an Unhealthy Diet

There are many definitions out there with regard to what unhealthy diets are. This section will explain what an unhealthy diet is by looking at the main components that characterize them. Let's get started!

Too Many Calories

First and foremost, we should clear the misconception that calories are completely unhealthy. The calories in your food provide your body with energy to help sustain your survival. Everything that you do on a daily basis derives energy from the calories from your diet. This means that calories are a necessity for survival. However, consuming too many calories negatively affects your health.

A diet that has a high-calorie content is unhealthy, especially when your lifestyle incorporates little to no physical activity. This implies that the exact calorie intake is different for every individual, depending on their body and activity levels. However, the general guidelines by the National Institutes of Health (NIH) stipulate that a female in their middle ages and with moderate activity should not eat more than 2,000 calories within a day. If you are male, your calorie intake should range between 2,400 and 2,600 calories each day (National Institutes of Health, 2013).

Foods that are high in processed sugar and saturated fats have high-calorie content. Such food has taken over the larger part of the diets of many communities, especially Western ones. High amounts of calories, coupled with low nutrient value, are also known as "empty calories."

Some of the high-calorie foods that you might be fond of are ice cream, doughnuts, french fries, chocolates, cookies, and other commercially available foods that are highly processed. For instance, a large cookie that is coated with chocolate harbors more than 220 calories in it (U. S. Department of Agriculture, 2020). A simple glazed doughnut is a home for more than 300 calories (Link, 2021). That's quite a lot!

High in Fat

Not all fats are bad for your health. However, there are some fats that you should be on the lookout for so that you limit their consumption as much as possible. For you to understand the types of fats that you should not eat, we will look at the different types of fats that exist.

- **Unsaturated fats:** This type of fat exists as a liquid under room temperatures. Unsaturated fats are further classified into two types which are monounsaturated and polyunsaturated fats. Foods such as avocados, peanuts, hazelnuts, as well as sesame and pumpkin seeds are rich in monounsaturated fats. Canola and olive oils are also added to this list. Examples of foods that contain high amounts of polyunsaturated fats are walnuts, fish, and soybean oil. Unsaturated fats are healthy. This is mainly because these fats improve cholesterol levels in your body when you eat them as part of your diet.
- **Trans-fats:** Trans-fats are usually vegetable oils that would have gone through a process of hydrogenation. Since hydrogenation hardens these fats, they exist as solids at room temperature. Margarine, cookies, salad dressings, and some snacks like chips are all examples of trans-fats. You should limit your consumption of trans-fats. They can significantly raise your cholesterol levels.

- **Saturated fats** are also referred to as "solid fats" because they are always solid at room temperatures. Saturated fats are usually found in animal foods like meat, milk, and cheese. Foods that have margarine as part of their ingredients because they are very easy to digest. Saturated fats are the most dangerous if you consume them in large amounts in your diet. They tend to increase bad cholesterol levels, also known as low-density lipoprotein (LDL) while reducing good cholesterol, also called high-density lipoprotein (HDL).

Excessive Sugar

Sugar is a carbohydrate. Other forms of carbohydrates are starches and fiber. Both of these are complex carbohydrates that take much time to digest. However, sugars are simple carbohydrates that can quickly flood the bloodstream with glucose immediately after eating them. Some of the foods rich in simple sugars include cookies, candy, doughnuts, sweet rolls, sugar-sweetened drinks, and dairy desserts like yogurt and ice cream.

Fad Diets

A fad diet is one that becomes popular for a limited period of time, for some reason. Some of them are created to answer specific 'needs' like weight loss. As a result, they tend to eliminate some crucial aspects of a healthy diet. For instance, some fad diets are made to enhance immediate weight loss, and so they will take out essential nutrients like carbohydrates. Remember, your body really needs these nutrients but in the right amounts. Completely eliminating any of them is not a good option.

Pointers for an Unhealthy Gut

A healthy gut is a must-have if you want your whole body to be sound, too. This is because your gastrointestinal tract influences other components of your body's health, your immune system included. Therefore, it is vital that you understand how you can detect an unhealthy gut so that you can take the right steps to alleviate any issues for the sake of your overall health. In this section, we will discuss various things that you should not take for granted if you experience them in your gut.

Increased Sweet Tooth

If your sugar cravings are more than usual, it's something to get worried about. Here is why. When you eat a lot of sugar as part of your diet, the number of beneficial bacteria in your gut can be reduced. If this happens, you will begin to feel like eating even more sugar. The more you succumb to this vicious cycle, the more you damage your gut even more.

Unplanned Weight Changes

When there is an imbalance in your digestive system, you might gain or lose weight without your intention. Some malfunctions in your gut compromise digestion and absorption processes. This, in turn, affects the types and amounts of nutrients that are available for use by your body. Your body becomes less able to control glucose. This might also affect your body's ability to store energy in the form of fat.

When this happens, the only way your body knows best to compensate for the nutrient shortage is by increasing food consumption. The moment you start eating more, the probability that you will gain weight will increase. You will even become more vulnerable to becoming obese.

Unusual Food Intolerances

You might have had some food intolerances that you were aware of in your life. In the event that you start noticing new signs of food intolerances, your gut might be involved. Generally, food intolerances are a sign that your digestive system is unable to digest certain foods. This might be attributed to the composition of the gut microbiota. If the quality of the bacteria in your gut is poor, there are some foods that you won't be able to digest. Food intolerances are usually characterized by symptoms such as diarrhea, nausea, pain, and bloating.

Sleep Disturbances Coupled With Chronic Fatigue

The hormone serotonin, which is predominantly produced in the gastrointestinal tract, governs your mood and sleep patterns. There is, therefore, no doubt that a gut whose health is compromised might contribute to sleep-related problems, especially insomnia, which is sleeplessness. If insomnia stretches for too long, it will result in chronic fatigue.

Unsettled Stomach

Please note that the activities that are enhanced by your gut microbiota as they act on food might release some gas. This is a normal process. However, excessive gas production should be a cause for concern as this may trigger heartburn and bloating. When excessive gas is released in your gut, you may also experience irritation and pain in your stomach. When such things happen, you should know that something is wrong in your gut. Diarrhea and constipation are also signs of an unsettled stomach.

Autoimmune Conditions

Remember, the health of your gut also contributes to your mental well-being. Your ability to manage stress can also be highly dependent on the health status of your gastrointestinal tract. Simply put, any imbalance in your gut can lead to mental discrepancies that promote mood-related disorders, such as depression, stress, and anxiety. A recent study reported that stress could lead to autoimmune conditions like rheumatoid arthritis (Shmerling, 2020).

Skin Irritation

If you are experiencing unusual irritation on your skin, the root of the problem might be in your digestive system. Imbalances in your gut can cause Skin-related conditions such as rosacea, acne, and eczema. Some food allergies and unhealthy diets may lead to inflammation in the gut, further causing protein leakages that should not happen—such leakages aid skin irritation.

You Can Help Your Gut!

Now that you understand how important your gut is to the proper functioning of your body and your well-being, it's vital that you learn to keep it healthy. You should keep it in a state that helps it to play its roles with limited to no hindrance at all. This requires your input for it to happen. This section is a compilation of ideas that assist you to create a better working environment for your gastrointestinal tract.

Reduce Levels of Stress

Stress is one of the major hindrances with regard to how your gut will function. With its effects on digestion and absorption, stress will eventually affect the rest of your body. Therefore, it is to the best of your overall health that you deal with stress appropriately so as to get it out of the way and promote good functioning of your gut.

It might be difficult to avoid getting stressed in the first place, but there is a lot that you can do to alleviate its effects on your body. Interventions such as meditation, yoga, exercising, diffusing essential oils, talking to someone, and getting enough sleep. Watch a movie or create an environment that will help you to laugh the stress out. Eating right is one of the easiest ways to deal with stress. Eat foods that enhance the growth of your gut microbiota so that more serotonin, which is the "happy hormone," is produced in your digestive system. Know yourself—if a cup of tea will wash down your stress, drink it!

Slow Down When Eating

There is no need to rush when eating. Take one reasonable bite at a time and chew it slowly and thoroughly before swallowing. This increases the efficiency of digestion and absorption processes, which start in the mouth. When you rush your eating, the food is not adequately mixed with digestive enzymes in the saliva. Poor digestion in the mouth may result in digestive discomfort, which you can avoid.

Consider Using Prebiotics or Probiotics

Your gut will benefit if you add probiotics or prebiotics to your diet. Probiotics are live bacteria that are beneficial to your body. Foods such as plant-based yogurt may have helpful bacteria that add to your gut microbiota. Probiotics are foods that the gut microorganisms can feed on as they grow, multiply, and carry out their functions. Fiber-rich foods are a great example of a prebiotic.

Please note that if you have conditions such as SIBO (small intestine bacterial overgrowth), which is characterized by an excess in bacterial growth, do not use probiotics because they might worsen your situation. Besides, not all probiotics really work. Therefore, consider approaching your doctor for advice on which probiotics really work for you.

Sleep Well

The quantity and quality of your sleep matter much when it comes to gut health. For an average adult, it is recommended that you have at least seven to eight hours of quality sleep. This helps to maintain a healthy environment for the microbial communities in your digestive system.

Assess the Presence of Food Intolerances

Signs such as diarrhea, cramping, nausea, abdominal pains, rashes, bloating, and acid reflux are pointers that you might be experiencing food intolerances. Determine which foods might be responsible for these symptoms. You can try stopping to eat certain foods that you suspect and see if there are any notable changes in the signs that are related to food intolerances. Once you have identified the exact foods that your body cannot tolerate, eliminate them from your diet. You will see desirable improvements in the way your gastrointestinal tract functions.

Keep Yourself Hydrated

Never underestimate the importance of drinking plenty of water. It does good not only to your gut but the whole body as well. Enough water in your body keeps the mucosal lining of your intestines healthy, thereby contributing to its efficiency. A well-hydrated body also assists you in maintaining a good balance of beneficial bacteria in your gut. Drinking water also comes in handy in reducing constipation. At least two liters each day will do your digestive system good.

Alter Your Diet

Change your diet by doing away with unhealthy foods like those with excessive amounts of fats and sugars. Instead, include more plant-based foods that are supportive of a healthy gut. Make sure your diet has all the essential nutrients in their correct amounts.

The "Must-Eat" Foods

The health of your gut is highly dependent on the types of foods that you eat. Eliminating fatty and sugary foods from your diet is very effective in enhancing the gut's proper and more efficient functioning. However, additional knowledge on the types of foods that you should eat is also an effective strategy for promoting a healthy gut. For this reason, this section will delve into the foods that are recommended for the betterment of your gastrointestinal tract.

- **Foods that are rich in fiber:** Make your diet as fiber-rich as possible. Some of the foods that you can include are peas, berries, legumes, leaks, oats, beans, and asparagus.
- **Fermented foods:** Fermented foods are excellent sources of probiotics. Examples of such foods include plant-based yogurt, kimchi, sauerkraut, miso, and tempeh.
- **Onion and garlic:** Apart from their anticancer properties, onion and garlic have properties that promote the healthy functioning of the immune system (Dix, 2020). With such attributes, garlic and onion can also protect your gastrointestinal tract from diseases and cancers.

A diet, especially a plant-based one, can really help you turn over a new leaf and obtain a healthier and more nutritious lifestyle. These diets come with incredible benefits, unlike the vast inconsistencies that are associated with unhealthy diets. So, how exactly does a plant-based diet work? Find out in the next chapter.

4

―――――

INTO THE SCIENCE OF A
PLANT-BASED DIET

Some people believe that vegetarianism or veganism is just a trend or a phase that people will forget sooner or later. In fact, the plant-based diet is growing in popularity because of the many benefits that come with it. In this chapter, you will learn about the science behind this healthy diet and what drives its popularity. We will also explore the different kinds of plant-based diets that exist in the world. Simply put, this chapter dives deeper into the nitty-gritty of what a plant-based diet is all about.

The Plant-Based Diet

A plant-based diet is hinged upon foods that are either plants or derived from them. Plant-based diets include limited to no animal-based products. Vegetables, fruits, seeds, legumes, whole grains, and nuts form the backbone of plant-based diets. Some use the terms plant-based and

39

vegan interchangeably. Such people believe that a plant-based diet is absolutely made up of plants and their products—no meat. However, to some, eating a 100% vegan diet does not define a plant-based diet. This group of people believes that plant-based foods dominate a plant-based diet, but it is still acceptable to eat some animal products here and there. We will discuss more on the different classifications of plant-based diets later in this chapter.

Plant-Based Diets and Nutrients

It is difficult to believe that you can have a highly nutritious diet without involving animal products. However, the truth is that most of the nutrients that your body needs are available in plants. In fact, most of the nutrients that animals have are derived from the plants that they eat. Carnivores eat some herbivores, so they still indirectly get the nutrients from plants.

It is also important to note that just the fact that a particular food is derived from plants doesn't necessarily make it healthy. There are other factors that you should consider. In one study, research revealed that participants who followed plant-based diets that were dominated by highly processed foods like refined grains were more prone to heart disease (Satija et al., 2017). In the same study, it was reported that participants whose diet was based on whole grains, legumes, fruits, vegetables, and nuts had a significantly reduced risk of suffering from heart disease. Therefore, more natural plant-based foods are healthy, but processed ones are not. The processing in the latter tends to remove a lot of the beneficial nutrients that the plants initially have.

Let's see some of the nutrients that you can get after eating components of a plant-based diet:

- **Proteins:** The moment you hear about this nutrient, it is easy to think of meat, eggs, and fish. Did you know that many plant-based foods are rich in proteins? Legumes like lentils, peas, beans, and chickpeas are excellent sources of proteins and amino acids. Not only these, some fermented plant-based foods like tempeh and tofu will also provide your body with proteins. Just a cup of tempeh has 33 grams of proteins embedded in it, while a three-ounce serving of tofu has eight grams (Byrne, 2019).
- **Vitamin B12:** Vitamin B12 is an essential vitamin that your body requires in very small amounts. However, if you get too little of the vitamin, you risk suffering from nerve damage, fatigue, and anemia. For vegans, the only way to get vitamin B12 is by eating fortified plant-based foods or taking supplements. Some of the most common vitamin B12 sources are soya yogurts, breakfast cereals, and plant-based dairy alternatives.
- **Iron and zinc:** If you need zinc and iron, you will never go wrong if you eat whole grains. This is especially true when they are not commercially processed. Iron and zinc are involved in various enzymatic processes in your body. Iron is also an important part of the hemoglobin that carries oxygen from your lungs throughout your body.
- **Calcium:** You need calcium for your bones. Cruciferous and leafy green vegetables are what you

need to get this nutrient without eating animal-based products. Sesame seeds and tempeh are other plant-based excellent sources of calcium.

- **Omega-3 polyunsaturated fats:** Although the richest source of omega-3 fatty acids is fish, you can still get this nutrient through a plant-based diet. Foods like flax seeds, hemp seeds, walnuts, and chia seeds contain essential fats that your body can convert to long-chain omega-3 polyunsaturated fatty acids. Oils from hemp, flaxseed, and rapeseed have remarkable amounts of essential omega-3 fatty acids.

Plant-Based Diet Categories

As we mentioned earlier, there is no "one-size-fits-all" way of describing plant-based diets. It all depends on what individuals believe. Here, we will classify people according to their take on what plant-based diets are. As you might notice, individuals in all the categories that we will describe have diets that have plants and their products as the backbone. Three only differ in their selection of animal-based foods.

- **Pescatarians:** In addition to other plant-based foods, pescatarians also eat shellfish and fish.
- **Lacto-vegetarians:** These people include dairy foods in their diet. Poultry, eggs, red meat, and seafood are not part of the list of what they eat.
- **Lacto-ovo vegetarians:** This group of individuals do not eat fish, red meat, or poultry. However, they eat animal products such as eggs and dairy foods.

- **Ovo-vegetarians:** Ovo-vegetarians shy away from dairy foods and other animal-based foods. They eat eggs, though.
- **Vegans:** This group completely stays away from animals and their products. They don't even eat dairy, eggs, and honey.
- **Semi-vegetarians:** Semi-vegetarians are also known as flexitarians due to their relative flexibility compared to other categories. They sometimes eat certain meats, as well as dairy, poultry, eggs, and seafood.

The Pros and Cons of a Plant-Based Diet

Like any other diet, plant-based diets come with their own advantages and disadvantages. Interestingly, the downsides of this diet are less than the benefits that are associated with this diet. This section will enlighten you on the pros and cons of the diet.

The Pros

Here are the advantages of a plant-based diet:

Amazing Health Benefits

There are numerous health benefits that come with eating plants and their products. These include

- **Heart health:** The more you eat plant-based foods, the lower the risk of heart-related diseases. Fruits, beans, nuts, whole grains, as well as substitutes for meat like soy reduce the probability of high bad cholesterol levels, high blood pressure, heart disease, and heart attacks. This was confirmed by recent studies (Choi et al., 2021). Bad cholesterol is capable of blocking your blood vessels, thereby increasing the chances of heart disease in the long run. Since plant-based foods increase good cholesterol levels, you are unlikely to have problems with your heart health if you eat them regularly.

- **Gut health:** Plant-based foods positively impact your gut microbiota in two ways. First, they can increase the number of bacteria that already exist in your gut. The microorganisms in your gut feed on these foods and multiply. Second, plant-based foods, especially those that are fiber-rich, may increase the diversity of the flora in your gastrointestinal tract. Some studies revealed that the incidences of colorectal cancers in vegans is 16% lower than in non-vegetarians (Wise, 2015). This shows that plant-based diets play a crucial role in promoting the health of the gut.

- **Lower risks of diabetes and obesity:** Plant-based foods take longer to get digested and pass through the gastrointestinal tract. This increases the time during which you feel satiated, thereby reducing unnecessary food consumption that might lead to obesity in the long run. The slower digestion of plant-based foods also comes with a steadier release of glucose into the bloodstream. This is contrary to what happens when you eat processed foods that can easily cause spikes in glucose levels in the bloodstream. When glucose is released at a slower rate, there is less room for it to be converted to fat for storage. Too much fat is the culprit for obesity. On the other hand, high glucose levels in the blood may trigger insulin resistance and cause diabetes.

Improved Overall Well-Being

Here are some of the things that plant-based foods can do for your overall well-being:

- **Increases your energy:** Apparently, plant-based foods are rich in complex carbohydrates and fiber. Fruits and vegetables also have lots of water. All this helps you to stay satiated for extended periods of time. As a result, you have a constant supply of energy for longer without you having to eat regularly. There are studies that even reported that plant-based diets could reduce fatigue (Plant-Based News, 2019).
- **Reduces aches and pains:** Research-based studies showed that diets that are based on plants can significantly reduce chronic pain (Towery et al., 2018). Plant-based diets are also attributed to enhancing quicker healing when you are injured. They also help to regulate inflammation levels.
- **Rejuvenates your mind:** If you want to enhance a healthier mind, plant-based diets are one of the options that you should consider. Swiss chard, spinach, kale, and other green leafy vegetables have

been experimented on (Morris et al., 2017). The results of the studies showed that they are effective in reducing cognitive decline. Foods that are plant-based also improve your memory, thereby making you smarter. Consuming plant-based foods that are rich in amino acids and short-chain omega-3 fatty acids can lower symptoms of depression, anxiety, and stress. Diseases like Alzheimer's disease can be prevented if your diet is rich in plant-based foods (Physicians Committee for Responsible Medicine, 2019).

Helps With Weight Loss

Research reveals that following a plant-based diet is an effective strategy toward achieving weight loss (Turner-McGrievy et al., 2015). There are many reasons why this is so. When you eat any type of food, glucose is absorbed into the bloodstream. Some of the glucose is converted to glycogen, which is stored in the muscles and liver. There is a limited amount of glucose that can be converted to glycogen at any given time. Therefore, if there is any excess glucose in the bloodstream after the glucose-to-glycogen conversion, it is then converted to fat as a form of energy storage. These fat stores significantly contribute to weight gain. So, unlike other foods, especially sugary and processed ones, plant-based foods are digested at a slower rate, so the glucose is steadily released into the bloodstream. This means that there isn't too much glucose in the blood at a given time. Alone, this is a stride toward weight loss.

The fact that plant-based foods are digested slowly also means that they stay in your gastrointestinal tract for longer. The positive effect of this is that you remain full for longer periods. This reduces the need to consume more food, some of which may cause spikes in glucose levels.

Plant-based foods improve the numbers and diversity of microorganisms in your gut. This improves digestion and absorption, making nutrients available for use by your body. Otherwise, your body will be deprived of the nutrients that it needs. To make up for this "fake deficiency" of nutrients, you will feel hungry and eat more than you should. This will aid weight gain. However, this scenario is less likely when you eat plant-based foods.

They are Less Restrictive

Unlike other types of diets, the plant-based diet is less restrictive. You don't need to worry about restricting portions and counting calories to remain healthy. Let's take it this way, weigh 300 calories of berries versus those of cookies. You will realize that a few cookies have the same number of calories as a large number of fruits. Do you see why counting calories is simply an unnecessary additional task when it comes to plant-based diets?

They Have Beneficial Compounds

Plant-based food harbors various beneficial compounds inside them. When you eat them, you also eat these compounds that are useful to the healthy functioning of your body. We mentioned some of the nutrients and vitamins that plants have earlier in this chapter. In addition to these, plants also contain compounds that are known as phytochemicals. These are plant-based compounds that often exhibit medicinal and pharmacological properties. Plants produce such compounds to protect themselves from diseases, pests, and even herbivores. However, extensive research revealed that phytochemicals also confer health benefits to humans. Phytochemicals can act in different ways in your body. Examples include

- **Antioxidant activity:** Antioxidants are compounds that are capable of scavenging free radicals that could trigger some diseases, like cancers. When your body carries out metabolism, free radicals are produced. Typically, your body has a robust antioxidant system that removes these oxidative radicals from your body. However, sometimes, the natural antioxidant system in your body is overpowered. This is why additional antioxidants from your diet are vital. Some plants contain phenolic compounds and flavonoids. These phytochemicals exhibit potent antioxidant activity. Green leafy vegetables are rich in polyphenolic compounds.
- **Lowering blood pressure:** Anthocyanins are involved in lowering your blood pressure. This keeps your heart healthy. To get anthocyanins, eat berries.
- **Anticancer activity:** Some phytochemicals have been identified for their anticancer activities (Rosewell Park, 2019). Lycopene and carotenoids are examples of such compounds. You can get

carotenoids and lycopene when you eat broccoli, carrots, orange squash, sweet potatoes, and cooked tomatoes.

Prevents Diseases

When you eat plant-based foods, you protect your body from exposure to some substances and chemicals that could harm it. Let's see some of the mechanisms of action through which the plant-based foods in your diet protect you:

- **Fighting chronic inflammatory diseases:** Inflammation is part of your body's response to fighting infection and diseases. In that regard, inflammation is a friend. However, when inflammation gets prolonged and chronic, it becomes an enemy. Chronic inflammation is often linked to other diseases like diabetes, Alzheimer's disease, depression, and arthritis. Plant-based diets offer the easiest way to deal with chronic inflammation. Tomatoes, spinach, walnuts, blueberries, almonds, oranges, kale, olive oil, and cherries are some of the food to keep in your house if you are targeting chronic inflammation.
- **Keeps chemical additives away:** Most plant-based foods are more natural and, therefore, lack possibly harmful chemical additives. Some of these additives increase the levels of oxidative free radicals in your body.

Contributes to the Environment

Eating plant-based diets is not only a benefit to humans. It is also advantageous to other components of the globe, including animals. Our environment also benefits when we make plants the main part of our diet. Here, we will discuss how the environment benefits when more people subscribe to plant-based diets.

- **Minimizes cruelty on animals:** Some regard killing animals for food to be cruel. The same applies to taking their products and eating them. For example, the milk from cattle is meant for their calves, so drinking this milk can be taken as cruelty to both the mother cow and its calf.
- **Protects the physical environment:** It is hypothesized that in the event of a global shift toward plant-based foods, the emission of greenhouse gasses as a result of food production might reduce by 70% by the time we reach 2050 (Physicians Committee for Responsible Medicine, n.d.). This is because the production of animal-based foods is associated with greater emissions of greenhouse gasses compared to plant-based products. This notion is especially true for methane and carbon dioxide.

Easier to Manage

It is often easier to prepare a plant-based meal than an animal-based one. The former is, therefore, less time-consuming and more readily available. Moreover, plant-based foods are generally less expensive than animal-based ones. This might be due to the complex processes that are involved in preparing animal products before they can be consumed.

The Cons

There are a few disadvantages that come with eating a plant-based diet. One of the main issues is that you might not be able to get enough nutrients as you would if you were incorporating animal-based diets, too. This applies to individuals who decide to exclude all animal products and stick to a completely plant-based eating style.

When you are on a plant-based diet, please pay special attention to your protein and vitamin intake. Vitamin B12 is one of the vitamins that are not readily available in plant foods. It is, therefore, important to know where you can get such vitamins — fortified foods will do. Also, check for minerals like iron and calcium because they might not be available in some plant-based foods. Some amino acids that are needed by your body are not available in plant-based foods. You can supplement some of these vitamins and minerals to enhance a more balanced plant-based diet.

The Evidence

The information that we have been providing you so far is hinged on results that were reported from scientific studies. In this section, we will briefly give you the evidence that supports various notions about plant-based diets. This will help you to determine the authenticity of the fact that plant-based diets are really good for your gut and overall health.

The Effects of Plant-Based Diets on Your Gastrointestinal Tract

The positive effects of vegetarian and vegan diets on your gut have been proved by research. Studies report that individuals who are on vegetarian and vegan diets have a variety of microorganisms growing in their gut, and this is an advantage (Glick-Bauer and Yeh, 2014). However, the diversity of the microbes in the guts of omnivores is limited. Some of the reasons that explain these differences in gut microbiota are substrate differences, pH, the general transit time of the food through the digestive system, and the types of microorganisms consumed in food.

There is a connection between microbial diversity in the gut and factors such as body mass index (BMI), arterial compliance, and obesity. Interestingly, plant-based diets do affect these factors in positive ways, thereby impacting the diversity of microorganisms in the gut. A study that was done by Natalia Klimenko and colleagues concluded that there is a positive correlation between microbial richness in the gut and long-term consumption of vegetables and fruits (Klimenko et al., 2014). The results from this study also confirmed the negative correlation between BMI and microbial diversity in the gut.

Plant-Based Food Components and the Gut Microbiota

Various components of plant-based foods exert different effects on the gut microbiota. One of such effects is that the nutrients in plants have a lower bioavailability. This means that releasing these nutrients from the plant-based food for absorption does not readily occur. Such a scenario allows more significant amounts of nutrients to reach the lower parts of the digestive system, where they can be made available to gut microorganisms (Ercolini and Fogliano, 2018). This way, plant-based foods support the development, growth, and functions of the gut microbiota. This also explains why ultra-processed foods and acellular nutrients that can be easily absorbed into the bloodstream are relatively less beneficial to the microorganisms in your gut.

Plants contain non-digestible carbohydrates like resistance starch. Such carbohydrates will successfully pass through the digestive system until they reach the large intestines. Here, they are fermented by the gut microorganisms to produce energy and postbiotics as products. Through scientific research, it has been determined that non-digestible carbohydrates increase the abundance of lactic acid bacteria like *Roseburia* and *Ruminococcus* while reducing the presence of *Enterococcus* and *Clostridium* species (Singh et al., 2017). Please note that digestible carbohydrates from fruits cut down the abundance of the *Enterococcus* and *Clostridium* species, too. Such carbohydrates include fructose, glucose, and sucrose.

Both the quality and quantity of the fats that you consume will impact your gut microbiota. Compared to an animal-based diet, a plant-based diet contains lower amounts of fats, which supports the development of *Bifidobacteria*, which are beneficial to your body. Here is another worthwhile mention —walnuts increase *Bifidobacteria* and *Ruminococcaceae* while decreasing *Clostridia* (Bamberger et al., 2016). This is a desirable scenario to create in your gut as it enhances better health for your gut and the rest of your body.

Effects of Diet on Gut and Overall Health

Sometimes, the term "gut microbiome" can be used in place of "gut microbiota" to describe the microorganisms that stay in your gut. We have seen how the various components in your diet are likely to affect your gut microbiome. Now, we will slightly shift our focus to the health impacts that these components have on your gut and the rest of your body.

Fats

Consuming saturated and trans fats increases the probability of you suffering from cardiovascular diseases. This is because these types of fats increase bad cholesterol (LDL cholesterol) levels in your blood and body. Contrastingly, unsaturated fats alleviate the risk of heart-related diseases. The better part of it all is that plant-based foods are good sources of unsaturated fats, making them relatively healthier.

Carbohydrates

While digestible carbohydrates in plants also have beneficial effects on health, the non-digestible ones are what make plant-based foods unique. Apart from the positive effects on the gut microbiota, non-digestible carbohydrates also reduce insulin resistance and chemicals that promote inflammation (Keim and Martin, 2014). Consuming non-digestible carbohydrates lowers the risk of obesity, too.

Proteins

Proteins in peas are reported to increase the levels of short-chain fatty acids (SCFA) in your intestines. Some studies have shown that these fatty acids have anti-inflammatory attributes (Kim et al., 2014). They are also involved in maintaining the mucosal barrier. Some of the microorganisms that are promoted by eating red meat are coupled with an increase in trimethylamine-N-oxide (TMAO). This compound elevates the risk of cardiovascular ailments (De Filippis et al., 2016). Too high intake of proteins, as is usually the case when you consume animal-based diets, increases the levels of insulin-like growth factor 1 (IGF-1), which is linked to elevated risks of diabetes, cancer, and overall mortality. Experimental work showed that plant-based proteins are associated with lower mortality. Simply put, proteins from plants are linked to an increased lifespan (Levine et al., 2014).

Probiotics

Fermented foods contain lactic acid bacteria. These microorganisms are ingestible as you consume fermented foods. This way, probiotics help to prevent inflammatory bowel disease, in addition to regulating the health of your intestines (Shen et al., 2014). Results from another study revealed that consuming probiotics increased the levels of good cholesterol (HDL cholesterol) and insulin sensitivity. Participants who did not take probiotics had lower HDL cholesterol levels and increased insulin sensitivity (Rajkumar et al., 2014). If you are showing food intolerance symptoms, fermented foods can help. Probiotics also improve your humoral immune response by increasing IgA in the serum (Link-Amstr et al., 1994).

A plant-based diet is not all that complicated. There are so many different ways through which it can help you to transition into a healthier lifestyle. The pros definitely outweigh the cons, and it has proven to be quite an effective diet. With all this evidence and research available out there, let's get into exactly what a plant-based diet can do for the mind and the body.

5

PLANT-BASED HEALTH

When it comes to a plant-based diet, we've looked at the pros, cons, details, evidence, and much more. We've seen what a plant-based diet can do for your gut and how a bad diet can truly mess up the processes of your gut, thereby deteriorating your health. This chapter will give you a better outlook on what a plant-based diet can do for you. It isn't just about a healthy gut but also a healthy mind and body. Having said this, let's take a deep look into the other benefits of a plant-based diet, from a healthy mind to a healthy body.

A Healthy Mind

While the brain on its own is a mystery, the effects that the plant-based diet has on this organ are not! Dr. Michael Grego, who is a clinical nutritionist and a fellow at the American College of Lifestyle Medicine, once said, "Plant-based eating can improve not only body weight, blood sugar levels, and ability to control cholesterol, but also emotional states, including depression, anxiety, fatigue, and sense of well-being, and daily functioning" (Debret, 2021). This section will enlighten you on the health effects of a plant-based diet on your mind.

Helps Your Brain to Age Gracefully

Normally, the functionalities of your brain tend to be less efficient as you age. This comes with some health conditions like Alzheimer's disease and dementia. A plant-based diet comes in handy when it comes to reducing your risk of suffering from these diseases. Another interesting fact that scientific experiments have shown is that the mind-body connection is crucial if you are to age healthily and happily. However, this mind-body link is gradually disrupted as you become older. You won't need to worry much about that if you incorporate more plant-based foods into your diet. Compounds in plant-based foods prevent inflammation that comes with aging. This diet also boosts your immune system, thereby maintaining or even improving your body's ability to fight infections and other triggers for diseases. Eating a plant-based diet is a worth-the-while investment for your retirement.

Improves Your Intelligence

Would you believe that diets that are based on plant-based foods make you smarter? Yes, this notion is based on findings from research. The first study of this kind was done in 1980 at Tufts University, and its results showed that the vegetarian children who participated in the study had IQs that were around 16 points above the average (Gregor, 2007).

Conclusions were also made that these children's "mental age" was one year further ahead compared to that of their classmates who were not vegetarians.

Another group of researchers working from the University of Southampton embarked on a study that involved 8,000 participants. This study spanned 20 years. The participants who were the brainiest were the ones who shunned fish and meat. This further supported the notion that plant-based diets positively contribute to your intelligence.

Betters Your Overall Mood

Individuals who eat plant-based diets are happier for the better part of their time. This is more so if they eat plant-based foods that are rich in amino acids and short-chain omega-3 fatty acids. These nutrients reduce the negative feelings that are associated with stress, anxiety, and depression. Please note that your plant-based diet does not replace mental health treatments and psychological therapies overseen and facilitated by health professionals. Adding a plant-based diet to these interventions will give you better results and lift your mood in a sustainable way.

Apart from omega-3 fatty acids, foods that will provide you with tryptophan will help. Tryptophan is an amino acid that is used by your brain to produce the "happy hormone," serotonin. While you can get this amino acid from fish, chicken, and cheese, there are plant-based sources for tryptophan. These include mushrooms, sunflower seeds, leafy greens, pumpkin seeds, broccoli, watercress, and peas.

B vitamin also boosts the production of serotonin in your brain. This way, it contributes to a less stressed spirit. Fortified cereals, legumes, and sunflower seeds are all great sources of B vitamins.

Dealing With Psychological Discrepancies

As mentioned earlier, eating vegetables, fruits, and grains is an inexpensive way to deal with psychological issues like depression and stress. Animal products like chicken and eggs contain arachidonic acid, which triggers chemical reactions that cause inflammation. The brain can be affected by this inflammation, leading to feelings of stress, anxiety, and/or depression. The easiest way to avoid arachidonic acid is by staying away from animal foods that are rich in the chemical. Eating more plant-based foods will help!

One study investigated the link between dietary patterns and depression (Akbaraly et al., 2009). The 3,486 participants who volunteered to take part in the study were assessed over a period of five years. It was noted that those who ate whole foods experienced fewer depression symptoms compared to those who consumed processed foods. This study showed that plant-based foods can contribute to alleviating symptoms of depression.

A Healthy Body

There are so many reasons to go on a plant-based diet. It doesn't have to be only about the gut because the diet has so many health benefits that can rejuvenate your body and make you feel new. Due to the advantages that come with plant-based diets, this eating pattern has become so popular. This section will delve deeper into other long-term benefits that a plant-based diet will give to your body.

Lower Blood Pressure

High blood pressure is also referred to as hypertension. This condition can trigger other diseases like type 2 diabetes, heart disease, stroke, and potentially a heart attack. If you have hypertension already, you can deal with it by watching what you consume every day. Shifting to a more plant-based diet is a step you can take to reduce blood pressure. Some studies revealed a 34% decrease in the chances of developing high blood pressure in vegetarians compared to non-vegetarians (Chuang et al., 2016). This is a significant decrease that can see you overcoming hypertension in the long run if you stick to your plant-based diet.

A Healthier Heart

The damage that can be made to the cardiovascular system by saturated fats cannot be underestimated. These fats can cause blockage in blood vessels, thereby compromising blood flow to and from different parts of the body. The pressure that is exerted on these blood vessels due to fatty blockages can even strain their walls and eventually cause deadly leakages. Saturated fats are available in abundance in meat. Therefore, doing away with meat is the way to go. You then have to replace the meat with plant-based proteins. Some researchers investigated the effects of plant-based diets on cardiovascular diseases (Kim et al., 2019). Their findings showed that plant-based diets reduced the risk of cardiovascular diseases in participants by 16% and reduced mortality by 31%.

Improved Cholesterol Levels

As highlighted earlier, fatty foods are a threat to the proper functioning of your heart. If you eat a diet that is rich in fat, you risk suffering from cardiovascular diseases like coronary artery disease, heart attack, and stroke. A diet that is lower in unhealthy fats is more likely to reduce this risk and enhance a healthier cardiovascular system. This is where a plant-based diet comes in. This diet can lower bad cholesterol levels by about 10 to 15%. Strict vegan diets can even reduce this type of cholesterol further, with an average of 25% (Ferdowsian and Barnard, 2009). Bad cholesterol is the one that promotes heart-related diseases.

Lower Risk of Cancer

With all the other health benefits linked to a plant-based diet, you would also wonder if it can protect you from cancer? Mind you; cancer is one of the most dreaded diseases worldwide due to the high mortality rates associated with it. In 2020, approximately 10 million people succumbed to different types of cancer (Sung et al., 2021).

According to information that is hinged on research, cancer could be prevented by engaging in a plant-based diet. Plants contain some cancer-protective nutrients. These include fiber, vitamins, and minerals. Phytochemicals such as polyphenols have been attributed to preventing cancer when they are consumed in plant-based foods. Seeds, grains, vegetables, nuts, and fruits are some of the foods that contain these anticancer agents. An article published by the *Cancer Management and Research* journal reviewed the information that supports the notion that plant foods have a role to play in reducing cancerous attacks. From this review, it was stipulated that plant-based anticancer agents can cut down the risk of some cancers by 10% (Lanou and Svenson, 2010). Although this is moderate, it might be all you need to keep yourself safe from cancers, depending on the risk factors that surround you.

Minimized Stroke

Discrepancies that are related to the cardiovascular system can sometimes lead to stroke. This is especially true for high blood pressure, heart disease, and high cholesterol levels. Other risk factors for stroke are drinking alcohol, smoking, and substance abuse. The interesting part is that half of the existing strokes can be prevented. One of the interventions that could see you bypass the chances of experiencing a stroke is eating a plant-based diet. Just eat the vegetables, whole grains, and fruits to protect yourself from possible strokes. Those who eat more of the natural, unprocessed plant-based foods lower the risk of stroke by about 21% (Hu et al., 2014).

Increased Lifespan

All the other health benefits that are conferred by a plant-based diet will ultimately lead to one thing, which is a longer lifespan. A healthier being overall is a requirement if you want to live longer. In other words, diseases reduce your chances of survival while increasing the risk of dying. A study that was published in the Journal of the American

Heart Association reported that mortality rates can be reduced by 25% if you eat a plant-based diet (Kim et al., 2019).

To ensure that changing to a plant-based diet works, be sure to eat plant-based foods that are healthy. For instance, remove processed plant-based foods from your diet. This is why it is important to know the nutrients that various plant-based foods contain. You eat with knowledge and understanding. So, do away with refined grains and load your diet with legumes, healthy oils, whole grains, vegetables, and fruits.

You see, plant-based diets have grown in popularity mainly because of the many health benefits that come with it—you can attest to that based on the evidence from research that has been provided. Therefore, it's about time you make the switch to help your body, mind, and gut function properly and to their fullest potential.

6

MAKING THE SWITCH TO PLANT-BASED DIET

Many people want to switch to a plant-based diet but tend to find it a bit difficult to make the transition super-fast. It can be really overwhelming when you decide to go through the process, especially during the first few days or weeks. Still, the more you remain focused, consistent, and persistent, the better your lifestyle will become. In this chapter, you will learn the basic steps that you need to take for you to get into a plant-based diet to improve your lifestyle for the sake of your gut and overall well-being.

Get Into the Mindset

The transition from any other diet to a plant-based one begins in your mind. Once your mindset is ready, you will be better prepared to go through the great moments and hurdles of making changes to the diet that you were used to. Therefore, you need to start thinking of preparing your brain for the plant-based diet. One way of preparing your mindset to change toward a plant-based diet is by learning more about plant-based eating to better understand what you are getting into. That's what this book is for.

Think deeply about the positive side of the transition and tell yourself why you are doing this. There is no need to use willpower and deprivation strategies—understand what you are doing and make the transition gradual, fun, and objective.

Know What You Want

What is your end goal here? There needs to be a real and important reason why you want to get into a plant-based diet. If you're reading this book, it means you want to have a healthy gut. Find that special reason that gives you the motivation that you need for you to overcome any hardships when you are making the transition. When you have that reason in your mind, believe me, it will become super easy to get to that end goal!

The Steps

Let's face it; you are not going to wake up the next day and completely change your life to incorporate a plant-based diet. You don't want to put your body into shock. A radical change overnight will definitely make it much harder for you to get it right. This section will discuss some steps that you can take to make your transition toward a plant-based diet as easy as possible. These steps allow your body the time to adjust to the changes that come with a plant-based diet.

Start Small and Make It Gradual

For a start, aim at cutting down animal-based foods, not totally eliminating them. If the dinner that you knew all along would have to include red meat or chicken, completely removing them at once can be so difficult. However, you could start by selecting a few days in a week during which you don't eat meat at all and then increase them with time. Another good strategy involves starting with the plant-based foods that you dearly love. You can then gradually add other plant-based foods as you go. If you intend to go completely vegan, start by aiming at increasing the portions of plant-based foods in your diet. This way, your mind will get time to adjust to reducing animal-based products and increasing plant-based ones.

Continue Your Research and Education

A plant-based diet is quite broad. Therefore, taking your time to learn more about this healthy diet is a worthwhile endeavor. Check your previous diet and see if there are things that you would want to change. You will certainly want to do away with large consumption of meaty products. Now, find out plant-based replacements for those foods. For instance, you can replace meat and chicken with protein-rich fermented foods like tempeh and tofu. Plant-based foods also provide you with fiber, so you hit two birds with one stone!

Set Your Meal Plan

Planning out your meals is an important component of the process of switching to a plant-based diet. Create meal plans that favor abundant consumption of plant-based foods and their products. You can add meals with meat once in a while until you are able to get away from them completely if need be. The recipes that are lined up later in this book will assist you to start planning your meals. Once your mind is well-prepared and your meals are well-planned, eliminating animal-based foods becomes easier than you think!

Stick to Some Familiar Plant-Based Flavors

While you might be focusing on promoting a healthier gut, make sure you are also giving your body what it is happy with. Take advantage of the plant-based flavors that you have always loved. This will make the transition more enjoyable. You can even imitate some animal-based flavors using plants. If you are a tacos fan, why not prepare them using a plant-based recipe?

Start Reducing Your Dairy Intake

Now, focus on gradually eliminating dairy foods. This will only be tough if you decide to make the transition overnight, not overtime. Begin by finding a plant-based replacement for cow milk. Coconut, almond, and oat milk are some of the great options you could consider. After this, your next step would be to find products that are plant-based as replacements for yogurt prior to targeting cheese. Finally, take out other dairy products like sour and whipped cream.

Stock Your Favorite, Healthy Plant-Based Foods

Now that you are aware of the foods that you would be

eating in your newly-adopted plant-based diet, it's time to stock them up. Fill your pantry with the foods that promote your transition and do away with those that will tempt you to look back. This is a smart move that helps you achieve your transition goals.

Continue for Life

If you feel that your journey through the transition to a plant-based diet was easy, congratulations! If not, the good thing is that you made it, no matter how difficult it might have been. What is important now is for you to ensure that the plant-based diet is a sustainable part of your lifestyle. Stick to it and enjoy the benefits!

As elucidated in this chapter, transitioning to a plant-based diet can be really easy when you take the right steps. Take these steps, get into the mindset, and change your life for the better! To help you make the transition easier, the next few chapters will give you a list of exciting and delicious recipes for breakfast, lunch, dinner, and snacks.

7

THE RECIPES—BREAKFAST

There is a common saying that goes, "breakfast is the most important meal of the day." Therefore, knowing what to eat at this time is very important, especially if you want to keep your gut healthy. In this section, we will share some tips on how you can go about having an exciting, delicious, and nutritious breakfast. Let's dig in and enjoy as we explore.

Orange French Toast

The orange combined with the cinnamon gives this version of french toast a healthy zing. Aquafaba is a unique ingredient that comes from soaking beans or legumes. It provides a good balance of starch and proteins for the gut and body.

Ingredients

- Unflavored, unsweetened plant-based milk (1½ cup)

- Almond flour (½ cup)
- Aquafaba (1 cup)
- Pure maple syrup (2 tablespoons)
- Ground cinnamon (¼ teaspoon)
- Salt (2 pinches)
- Orange zest (½ tablespoon)
- Bread slices which are whole grain (3-inch size)
- Thawed, fresh, or frozen raspberries or blueberries (1 cup)
- Applesauce (½ cup)
- Pure maple syrup (1 teaspoon)

Steps

1. Mix plant milk, aquafaba, flour, salt, maple syrup, and cinnamon. Combine these ingredients until you create a smooth paste before transferring them to a shallow pan. Add the zest in and stir thoroughly.
2. Put a wire rake above a baking sheet, then preheat the oven to 400 °F.
3. Use a non-stick skillet that is warm on medium heat. Immerse each slice of bread into the mixture and leave it to soak for a few seconds. Please turn to the other side and allow it to soak as well. Place the well-soaked slice in the skillet for two to three minutes. Do the same on the other side until the whole slice appears golden brown.
4. Put the toasted bread onto the wire rake and bake in the oven for 10 to 15 minutes. Remove when it's crispy.
5. Now, for the final touch, take the applesauce and

maple syrup and place them in a blender. Process these until the sauce gives out a chunky consistency.

6. Take the toasted bread and spread the sauce onto it. Serve and enjoy! (Forks Over Knives, 2017)

Banana Smoothie With Vanilla

This meal will kickstart your day as it boosts your energy levels. Not only is it tasty, but it is also nutritious and unique. The banana smoothie with vanilla is packed with minerals, vitamins, healthy fats, and dietary fiber.

Ingredients

- Brewed chai tea (1 cup)
- Hemp seeds (2 tablespoons)
- Unsweetened plant-based milk (1 cup)
- Vanilla extract (½ teaspoon)
- Frozen banana (2 medium)
- Unsweetened plant-based butter (2 tablespoons)
- Avocado chunks (½ cup)
- Chia seeds (2 tablespoons)
- Vanilla protein powder
- Ice cubes (4)

Steps

1. Soak the chai tea for about five minutes.
2. Squeeze the extra tea which is in the bag and discard the residue.

3. Place all ingredients in a blender.
4. Finally, pour in some plant-based milk and all the other smoothie ingredients.
5. Serve your smoothie in a chilled glass while cold (Walder, 2020).

Gluten-Free Coconut Pancakes With Chocolate Chips

These pancakes are gluten-free and are laced with a chocolate chip flavor. They are filling and have healthy ingredients. You will enjoy your meal in just 30 minutes!

Ingredients

- Buckwheat flour (1 ¼ cups)
- Flaxseed meal (1 tablespoon)
- Unsweetened coconut flakes (2 tablespoons)
- Gluten-free rolled oats (¼ cup)
- Sodium-free baking powder or (1 tablespoon)
- Sea salt (1 pinch)
- Unflavored, unsweetened plant-based milk (1 cup)
- Unsweetened applesauce (½ cup)
- Pure maple syrup (¼ cup)
- Pure vanilla extract (1 teaspoon)
- Gluten-free, vegan mini chocolate chips (½ cup)
- Large, sliced banana (1)

Steps

1. Start by mixing the flaxseed with a half cup of water

in a small pot. Stir the mixture for three to five minutes on medium heat until it has a stringy consistency that allows it to drip from the spoon easily. Once the mixture is ready, remove the solids.

2. Take the applesauce, maple syrup, plant-based milk, vanilla, and flaxseed juice that you prepared in (1) above and pour these into the flour. Mix well. Make sure the batter is nice and thick before adding the chocolate chips.

3. Take a non-stick frying pan and place it over medium-low heat. While waiting for the pan to heat, measure a three-quarter cup of batter.

4. Carefully place the batter into the frying pan and cook until it is golden brown. Repeat this on the other side of the batter.

5. Follow steps three and four for the rest of the batter until it is finished.

6. Serve warm together with sliced banana, or add some maple syrup on top (Thacker, 2020).

Banana Almond Granola

This unique, delicious treat will keep you fuller for longer. It is a natural source of energy and is good for maintaining blood sugar levels. Another thing to note is that banana almond granola also lowers bad cholesterol levels.

Ingredients

- Rolled oats (8 cups)
- Pitted and chopped dates (2 cups)

- Peeled and chopped ripe bananas (2)
- Almond extract (1 teaspoon)
- Salt (1 teaspoon)
- Toasted, slivered almonds (1 cup)

Steps

1. As you heat your oven to 275 °F, get your oats and put them in a bowl.
2. Pour one cup of water into a pot until it boils, and maintain it on medium heat.
3. Throw the dates into the boiling water and leave them for 10 minutes. Monitor the dates, so they don't stick to the pot by consistently adding some water.
4. Take two baking sheets and line them with parchment paper whose measurements are 13 by 18 inches.
5. Place the mixture in a blender together with some almond extract, salt, and bananas. Aim for a smooth consistency.
6. Combine the date mixture and the oats prior to stirring thoroughly.
7. Separate the granola between the two baking sheets prepared earlier and spread evenly.
8. Bake for not more than 50 minutes. Be sure to stir at 10-minute intervals until the granola gets a crispy feel.
9. Take away from the oven and allow it to cool down before adding the slivered almonds.
10. Pack the granola in an air-tight container until you

need them. Serve in a small bowl with dates or raisins (Sroufe, 2015).

Chickpea Egg-Free Omelette

This is a simple recipe that takes 30 minutes to prepare. It is tasteful and adds nutritional value to your gut as it helps with healthy bowel movements.

Ingredients

- White pepper (¼ teaspoon)
- Black pepper (¼ teaspoon)
- Chickpea flour (1 cup)
- Nutritional yeast (⅓ cup)
- Baking soda (½ teaspoon)
- Green onions – white and green parts chopped (3)
- Sautéed mushrooms (4 ounces)
- Onion powder (½ teaspoon)
- Tomatoes, salsa, hot sauce, spinach, and microgreens (optional)
- Garlic powder (½ teaspoon)

Steps

1. Add all the dry ingredients: chickpea flour, white pepper, garlic powder, onion powder, black pepper, nutritional yeast, and baking soda in a bowl.
2. Pour in a cup of water to make a smooth batter.
3. Get a pan ready by heating it on medium heat.
4. Measure a three-quarter cup of batter and add to

the hot pan and cook. While cooking, add about two tablespoons of mushrooms and green onions to the batter to enhance the flavor.

5. Cook until the batter is golden brown before flipping to the other side.
6. To serve, place the omelet on serving plates, along with spinach, salsa, and hot sauce (Forks Over Knives, 2015).

Zucchini Bread With Steel Cut Oatmeal

This recipe is an excellent way of adding vegetables to your breakfast. This meal is gluten-free. You can even add some plain plant-based yogurt to increase its protein content. Antioxidants are also found in zucchini, and this makes it helpful in scavenging oxidative free radicals in your body.

Ingredients

- Ground cinnamon (½ teaspoon)
- Steel-cut oats (1 cup)
- Chia seeds (¼ cup)
- Vanilla extract (½ teaspoon)
- Grated zucchini (1 cup)
- Unsweetened, plant-based milk or water (2 cups)
- Toppings (walnuts, nut butter, maple syrup, and chocolate chips)

Steps

1. Use a grater to prepare the zucchini.

2. Put chia seeds, the prepared zucchini, and ground cinnamon in a saucepan and mix the ingredients.

3. Add the liquids, the plant-based milk and vanilla extract, over the steel cut oats.

4. Allow the oats to boil while occasionally stirring as you add in zucchini.

5. Reduce the heat as it simmers for approximately 17 minutes to allow the water to dry up.

6. To add sweetness, drizzle chocolate chips, maple syrup, or any of the toppings. Serve the oats in a small bowl as desired (Walder, 2020).

Polenta with Cranberries and Pears

This is a warm, filling recipe that will keep you going for the whole morning. In just 15 minutes, your meal will be ready! Use ripest pears and fresh cranberries to add to the flavor and nourishment. You will certainly not regret the effort.

Ingredients

- Ground cinnamon (1 teaspoon)
- Fresh or dried cranberries (1 cup)
- Brown rice syrup (¼ cup)
- Warm basic Polenta (1 batch)
- Peeled, cored, and diced pears (2)

Steps

1. Place the pot on a medium heat stove plate and add the rice syrup.

2. Put the pears, cinnamon, and cranberries into the rice syrup.

3. Cook, while occasionally mixing for 10 minutes.

4. Ready to serve! Put a touch of pear compote in each bowl (Sroufe, 2015).

Baked Oatmeal With Banana

This is a very rich recipe with oats that manage cholesterol levels in your body. The baked oatmeal with banana is a wholesome and filling recipe with healthy ingredients. You can think of the recipe as vegan baked oatmeal.

Ingredients

- Pecan pieces (1/2 cup)
- Rolled oats (2 cups)
- Cinnamon (1 ½ teaspoons)
- Allspice (1/2 teaspoon)
- Kosher salt (1/2 teaspoon)
- Baking powder (1 teaspoon)
- Plant-based milk (1¾ quarter cup)
- Ripe bananas (2)
- Pure vanilla extract (1 tablespoon)
- Banana slices, peanut butter, or almond butter
- Pure maple syrup (¼ cup)

Steps

1. Prepare an eight-by-eight pan by oiling it using a natural oil. Coconut oil will also do.

2. Startup the oven and let it heat to 375°F.

3. Put rolled oats, pecan pieces, baking powder, allspice, kosher salt, and cinnamon in a bowl before transferring them into the oiled pan.

4. Crush the bananas in a bowl and mix them with vanilla, maple syrup, and plant-based milk.

5. Now, gently sprinkle the plant-based milk mixture on the oats, making sure all ingredients are evenly fused.

6. Finally, place the prepared oats in the oven for about 40 to 45 minutes. The upper part should attain a golden color.

7. Take away from the oven and give your oats 10 minutes to cool down.

8. To add the icing to the oatmeal cake, put almond butter or peanut butter and spread it well.

9. Serve and garnish with banana slices (Overhiser, 2020).

Oatmeal with Fruits and Nuts

This is a quick recipe to prepare. When serving, add fruit or have it plain, as desired. There are a lot of varieties of fruits in the recipe, making it a good source of vitamins.

Ingredients

- Walnuts, pecans, chopped nuts, and cashews (2 tablespoons)
- Ground cinnamon (¼ teaspoon)
- Sea salt (1 pinch)

- Rolled oats (3¼ cup)
- Fresh berries (¼ cup) optional
- Sliced ripe banana
- Apricots (optional)
- Dried fruits, raisins, chopped apples, and raisins (2 tablespoons)
- Maple syrup

Steps

1. Add the oats and half a cup of water to a pot.
2. Allow the mixture to boil over high heat.
3. Lower the heat to medium or low intensity and cook for about five minutes until the water is finished.
4. Add fruits like berries, nuts, bananas, and some syrup to complete the dish.
5. Add cinnamon and salt upon serving (Sroufe, 2018).

Egyptian Breakfast With Beans

This is a high-protein recipe. Allow the beans to soak overnight. The recipe is good for the gut as it promotes the growth of beneficial gut bacteria and reduces cholesterol levels.

Ingredients

- Lemon zest and juice (1)
- Peeled medium yellow onion (1)
- Ground cumin (1 teaspoon)
- Dried and soaked fava beans (1½ pounds)

- Sea salt
- Quartered lemon (1)
- Peeled and minced garlic (4 cloves)

Steps

1. Wash the beans and remove the water. Add the beans to a saucepan.
2. Pour some water into the saucepan and allow the beans to boil over high heat.
3. Reduce the heat to medium heat so that the beans are slowly cooked for about two hours.
4. Fry onions in a different pot or saucepan on medium heat for not more than 10 minutes. When the onions almost become brown, throw in the lemon zest, garlic, cumin, lemon zest, and juice. Allow these to simmer for five more minutes.
5. Now, combine the beans and onion mixture and add some salt to taste.
6. To serve, put in a bowl and add some lemon quarters (Sroufe, 2016).

Apple Lemon Breakfast Bowl

This recipe has health benefits that are necessary to the gut. You are unlikely to have glucose spikes after eating this meal. Ground cinnamon slows the breaking down of carbohydrates in the gut, giving a balance of nutrients.

Ingredients

- Lemon juice (3 tablespoons)
- Medium-sized apples (5)
- Walnuts (2 tablespoons)
- Pitted dates (6)

Steps

1. Using a food processor, process half of the walnuts, lemon juice, cinnamon, and dates using a food processor until they are finely ground.
2. Prepare the apples by removing their seeds before adding them to the mixture in the food processor.
3. Add the other half of the apples and lemon juice to the processor and pulse till the apples are soft and the dates are evenly spread in the mixture.
4. Serve in a bowl with your favorite fruits with raisins or as desired (Karlsen, 2017).

Vegan Banana French Toast

The vegan recipe will assist in maintaining a healthy gut. Chia seeds help to clean the gut. The combination of the ingredients in this recipe creates a filling meal.

Ingredients

The French toast:

- Medium banana (1 ripe)
- Pure maple syrup (2 tablespoons)
- Unsweetened plant-based milk (1 cup)
- Chia seeds (1 tablespoon)

- Vanilla extract (1 teaspoon)
- Ground cinnamon (1 teaspoon)
- Gluten-free sandwich bread (8 slices)
- Coconut oil (¼ cup and 2 tablespoons)
- Kosher salt (¼ teaspoon)

For caramelized bananas:

- Diagonally sliced medium bananas (2)
- Coconut sugar (¼ cup)

To serve:

- Crushed raw pecans (2 tablespoons)
- Pure maple syrup
- Peanut butter or almond butter (not compulsory)

Steps

To make the french toast:

1. Switch on the oven to a low temperature that is not too hot.
2. Mix the maple syrup, chia seeds, banana, plant-based milk, cinnamon, vanilla, and salt in a blender until adequately mixed.
3. Leave the mixture in a dish to allow it to thicken.
4. To soak the bread, place it in the dish with the mixture for about 10 seconds. Turn it and do the same to the other side.

5. Take a saucepan and put some coconut oil to cook the soaked bread over medium heat.

6. Fry the bread for four to six minutes on each side until it turns golden brown and crispy on the edges. Add more coconut oil after flipping the bread.

7. To remove the excess oil, transfer the cooked french toast to a lined baking sheet and put it in the oven so that they also remain warm.

Making the caramelized bananas:

1. As you work on the French toast, mix the banana slices with the coconut sugar in a sealable plastic bag and let the ingredients be evenly covered with the coconut sugar.

2. To caramelize the banana, fry them in coconut oil for about two minutes.

3. To serve, put two slices of French toast on the plates and fairly share the pecans and caramelized bananas on top of the bread.

4. Almond butter, maple syrup, and peanut butter will add an extra delicious touch to the French toast (Overhiser, 2018).

Maple Pecan Muesli

This recipe is naturally gluten-free and contains proteins, unsaturated fats, and fiber that keep you full longer. Your gut microbiota also benefits from the fiber in this recipe.

Ingredients

- Unsweetened, non-shredded large coconut flakes (1 cup)
- Rolled oats (4 cups)
- Dried tart cherries (1 cup)
- Pecan pieces (1 ½ cups)
- Cinnamon (1 ½ teaspoons)
- Pure maple syrup and more to serve (2 tablespoons)
- Vanilla extract (2 teaspoons)
- Plant-based milk
- Nutmeg (⅛ teaspoon)

Steps

1. To prepare the dried cherries, chop them and put them aside in a bowl.
2. Switch on the oven to a temperature of 350°F.
3. Get another bowl in which you should mix the vanilla and maple syrup before putting them in a microwave for around 20 seconds. Also, combine coconut, spices, toasted oats, maple mixture, and pecans with the cherries in a bowl.
4. Put the mixture onto the baking sheet and dry it.
5. Place the oats evenly on a baking sheet, then spread the coconut in a layer on top.
6. Take another baking sheet and add the pecan pieces. Set the timer on and bake the contents on both trays for 10 minutes. The coconut should turn golden brown. Take the trays out of the tray and let them cool a bit.
7. When ready, pour over plant-based milk and add a bit of maple syrup.

8. Serve with desired fruits in a small bowl (Overhiser, 2017).

Chia Seed Pudding

The chia seed has omega-3 fatty acids that reduce inflammation. Fiber is also present that helps in bowel movements and lowering cholesterol.

Ingredients

- Pure maple syrup (1 tablespoon)
- Chia seeds (½ cup)
- Vanilla extract (½ teaspoon)
- Unsweetened plant-based milk (2 cups)
- Your choice of fruit or sliced raw almonds

Steps

1. Add plant-based milk, chia seeds, vanilla, and syrup in a bowl.
2. To show that the mixture is combining well, the consistency will thicken.
3. Serve in small bowls and add your sliced desired fruit (Donahue, n.d.).

Plant-Based Oatmeal Muffins

This is a very natural meal that gives high energy. These muffins will leave the gut feeling lighter yet full. This is all in one breakfast!

Ingredients

- Rolled oats (2 cups)
- Ground flaxseed (¼ cup)
- Walnuts (½ cup)
- Raisins (½ cup)
- Hot water (½ cup)
- Sea salt (¼ teaspoon)
- Maple syrup (¼ cup)
- Baking soda (¼ teaspoon)
- Cinnamon (2 tablespoons)
- Plant-based milk (½ cup)
- Banana (1)
- Apple (1)

Steps

1. Combine flaxseed with water and leave it for five minutes.
2. Mix all ingredients, including the flax mixture, in a food processor and run until well-combined. This should take about 30 seconds. Do not expect a smooth consistency.
3. When the batter is ready, put it in cupcake liners in a muffin tin and bake for 20 minutes at 350°F.
4. Serve with a hot cup of tea or chilled juice (Fawley, n.d.).

Black Bean Avocado Toast

The black bean avocado toast is a high-protein recipe that is mixed with corn for starch. This will keep you going until lunchtime with high energy. Black beans also prevent constipation. The avocado has high fiber, which is essential for proper digestion.

Ingredients

- Black beans (1 can)
- Chipotle spice (¼ teaspoon)
- Whole-wheat toast (2 pieces)
- Sea salt (a pinch)
- Black pepper (a pinch)
- Garlic powder (1 teaspoon)
- Juiced lime (1)
- Diced avocado (1)
- Corn (½ cup)
- Diced tomato (½)
- Fresh cilantro (a few tablespoons)
- Finely chopped red onions (3 tablespoons)

Steps

1. Combine cilantro, avocado, red onion, corn, tomato, the juice from half a lime, as well as a touch of salt and pepper in a bowl.
2. Combine beans, garlic powder, chipotle spice, a pinch of sea salt, and lime juice. Boil these

ingredients for 15 minutes to achieve a thick and starchy consistency.

3. Get four pieces of whole wheat bread and toast them.
4. Put the black bean mixture onto the toast when the toast is made.
5. Finish with the avocado mixture.
6. Serve with juice or tea (Fawley, n.d.-b).

8

———

THE RECIPES—LUNCH

After having your breakfast, you will definitely need to consider having a nutritious, plant-based lunch! This chapter delves into various dishes you can consider for a plant-based lunch. We will also provide you with step-by-step procedures for preparing them.

Tex-Mex Pita Pizzas

This is one of the best and easy homemade pizzas. It is topped with a black bean combo and tasty corn. This pizza is good for both kids and adults.

Ingredients

- Ground cumin (½ teaspoons)
- Minced garlic (2 cloves)
- Frozen or fresh corn kernels (1 cup)

- Chopped onion (1)
- Chopped avocado (1 cup)
- Pita rounds, whole wheat (6-7 inches)
- Oil-free salsa (1 cup)
- Snipped fresh cilantro (2 tablespoons)
- Rinsed and drained black beans (1 15-ounce can)
- Chopped bell pepper (1 cup)

Steps

1. Use parchment paper to line two clean baking sheets. While you do so, switch your oven and let it heat to 350°F.
2. Put the pita rounds on the baking sheets you prepared until they appear lightly roasted. This might take between 10 to 15 minutes.
3. Boil a quarter cup of water in a saucepan before adding garlic, cumin, and sweet pepper. Place the saucepan over medium to low heat for about 10 minutes. Be sure to add a few drops of water each time, coupled with occasional stirring to avoid sticking. Add the corn and beans, then cook for five minutes while stirring to ensure a consistent mixture of flavors. Make sure the corn and beans are well cooked.
4. Mash the avocado and spread it together with pita rounds and the bean mixture. Use salsa to top, then sprinkle with cilantro (Forks Over Knives, 2018).

Buddha Bowl

The vegan Buddha bowl is packed with nutrients. The beans, sauerkraut, fresh veggies, and turmeric tahini sauce makes this meal delicious and appetizing.

Ingredients

- Big cubed sweet potato (1)
- Quinoa or cooked brown rice (2 cups)
- Medium-sized carrots (2)
- Red radishes (2)
- Turmeric Tahini Sauce
- Cooked lentils or chickpeas (1 cup)
- Extra virgin olive oil
- Shredded red cabbage- (1 cup)
- Lemon (1 squeeze)
- Chopped kale (8 leaves)
- Fermented veggies (¾ cup)
- Microgreens
- Hemp or sesame seeds (2 tablespoons)
- Freshly cracked black pepper
- Sea salt

Steps

1. Line your baking sheet using parchment paper while you preheat the oven to 400°F.
2. Using olive oil, salt, and pepper, toss the sweet

potatoes before spreading them onto the lined baking sheet.

3. Peel the carrots into ribbons using a vegetable peeler and thinly slice the radish into rounds. A mandoline works best!

4. Squeeze the lemon and use it to toss the carrots, shredded cabbage, and radish slices. Set these aside.

5. Put the kale leaves into a bowl, then toss with a few pinches of salt and squeezed lemon. Massage the kale leaves with your hands until they decrease quantity in the bowl by about a half.

6. Bring together individual bowls with chickpeas, carrots, kale, microgreens radishes, sauerkraut, sesame seeds, cabbage, sweet potatoes, and brown rice. Use salt and pepper to season these dishes and serve them together with the Turmeric Tahini Sauce (Love and Lemons, 2017).

Chickpea Sandwich

The chickpea sandwich can be an excellent option for easy lunches throughout the week. It provides a great deal of fiber as well as protein to keep you full. This sandwich gets tons of flavor from fresh herbs.

Ingredients

- Plant-based yogurt (¼ cup)
- Basil leaves (¼ cup)
- Vegan mayonnaise (¼ cup)
- Diced celery (¼ cup)

- Salt
- Parsley leaves (¼ cup)
- Shredded carrots (¼ cup)
- Lemon zest (1 teaspoon)
- Lemon juice (2 tablespoons)
- Chickpeas (1 15-ounce can)
- Toasted bread (4 slices)

Steps

1. Transfer parsley, basil, plant-based yogurt, lemon zest, lemon juice, and vegan mayonnaise in a blender and process.
2. Add celery, carrots, and chickpeas to the mixture in (1) above and pulse not more than five times until the mixture is smooth but still chunky.
3. Put salt to taste before you add the mixture to two sandwiches. Enjoy! (Liz, 2018)

Collard Green Spring Rolls

This is a nourishing and healthy plant-based side or snack.

Ingredients

Spring rolls

- Extra-firm tofu (10)
- Collard seeds (1 bundle)
- Vertically thin-sliced small red bell pepper (1)
- Bean sprouts (1½ cups)
- Packed basil (1 cup)

- Finely sliced purple or red cabbage (1 cup)
- Finely chopped and peeled medium carrots (3)

Sauce

- Unsalted and creamy sunflower seed butter (1/3 cup)
- Tamari (2 tablespoons)
- Maple syrup (3 tablespoons)
- Juiced medium lime (½ lime)
- Thai red chili minced (1)
- Hot water

Steps

1. Chop off the stems of the collard greens and trim down the thickness of the stem at its base using a sharp knife. This will permit it to fold more easily.
2. Using an absorbent and clean towel, wrap your tofu. Set anything heavy on top of the wrap in order to drain any excess liquid.
3. Prepare the dipping sauce by mixing tamari, sunflower seed butter, lime juice, maple syrup, and chili garlic sauce in a bowl, then whisk to combine the ingredients. Adjust the viscosity of the sauce by adding hot water while whisking. The sauce should be pourable. Adjust the taste and flavors to match your preferences.
4. Slice the tofu into long, rectangular cubes, then arrange the pieces on a flat surface. Prepare the vegetables.
5. Lay a collard green on a flat surface and carefully

put basil, tofu, cabbage, carrot, bean sprout, and red pepper on top of it. Fold the collard green over once to cover the fillings inside. Carefully tuck them in the sides of the collard green and continuously roll until you have a spring roll that is loose. Make sure the seam side is facing down and set aside. Do the same for all the remaining fillings.

6. Slice the rolls into half or leave them whole, depending on your preference. Arrange the rolls in a serving bowl with the dipping sauce to serve (Minimalist Baker, 2017).

Lentil Vegetable Soup

This lentil soup is great for lunch and easy to make. The advantage of this soup is that it is flexible. For instance, if you don't have an ingredient, be it spinach or carrot, substitute with any of your favorite ingredients, or better still, just skip it.

Ingredients

- Finely chopped spinach (1-2 cups)
- Finely chopped carrots (2)
- Finely chopped small white potatoes (6)
- Water or vegetable broth (8 cups)
- Pepper and salt
- Finely chopped small onions (2)
- Brown lentils (1 16-ounce bag)
- Diced, fire-roasted tomatoes (1 15.5-ounce can)

Steps

1. Combine all ingredients but leave out the spinach.
2. Cook these ingredients on low heat for two hours.
3. Add spinach and cook for about 5 minutes before the soup is ready—season with salt and pepper to taste (McDougall, 2014).

Creamy Wild Rice Soup

Not only is the dark brown grains of the wild rice rich in nutrients, but they are also gluten-free. The chowder-style soup exudes the hearty goodness of wild rice!

Ingredients

- Trimmed and quartered button mushroom (1 8-ounce package)
- Vegetable stock (4 cups)
- Wild rice, uncooked, rinsed, and drained (¾ cup)
- Minced garlic cloves (4)
- Sea salt (¼ teaspoon)
- Chopped red bell pepper (1 cup)
- Almond flour (¼ cup)
- Thinly sliced leek (½ cup)
- Chickpea flour (¼ cup)
- White wine vinegar (1 tablespoon)
- Snipped fresh thyme (1 tablespoon)
- Chopped carrot (½ cup)

Steps

1. Add mushrooms, stock, garlic, wild rice, and leek in a soup pot. Boil with high heat, then reduce the heat to medium or low. Cover the pot and allow the contents to simmer for not more than 50 minutes. The kernels of the rice will start to pop open by then.
2. Add the bell peppers, salt, and carrots into the rice pot while stirring gently. Cover with a lid again and leave the contents to simmer for eight more minutes.
3. In a small bowl, bring together the chickpea and almond flours. Add a quarter cup of water and stir. Cook for a further two minutes while stirring. Until you achieve a bubbly and thick consistency, add another half cup of water before stirring in the vinegar and thyme (Christian, 2018).
4. Enjoy!

Roasted Veggie Grain Bowl

This is a rich recipe with profound variety in its ingredients. This grain bowl recipe contains lots of veggies, a scoop of sauerkraut, a vibrant sauce, and plant-based protein! The roasted veggie grain bowl is a "must-have" in your list of recipes!

Ingredients

- Raw and shelled pistachios/pepitas (½ cup)
- Chopped kale (1 packed cup)
- Small garlic (2 cloves)

- Fresh lemon juice (½ cup)
- Cilantro (1 cup)
- Freshly ground black pepper
- Water (3 cups)
- Extra virgin olive oil (½ cup)
- Sea salt (½ teaspoon)
- Honey/maple syrup (½ teaspoon)
- Rinsed raw quinoa (1 cup)
- Halved Brussels sprouts (1 ½ cups)
- Chopped parsnips (2)
- Broccolini (½ bunch)
- Florets from ½ cauliflower
- Sauerkraut (1 scoop)
- Drained and rinsed chickpeas (1 14-ounce can)
- Toasted pepitas (1 sprinkle)

Steps

1. Heat the oven beforehand to 425 °F. Using parchment paper, line two baking sheets.
2. Make the sauce by combining your kale, pepitas, cilantro, lemon juice, sea salt, olive oil, pepper, honey/maple syrup, garlic, and water in a blender. Process until the mixture is smooth.
3. Add rinsed quinoa to a pot and let it boil. Cover the pot with a lid and reduce the heat. Simmer for 15 minutes. Remove heat and allow it to sit while covered for ten more minutes.
4. Put the Brussels sprouts, cauliflower, and parsnips on one huge baking sheet and the Broccolini on the second baking sheet. Roast these vegetables until

they are golden brown on the edges. This might take about 25 minutes. Roast the Broccolini for about 12 minutes until it's tender. Drizzle some olive oil on the vegetables. Add pepper and pinches of salt, then toss to coat.

5. Combine the roasted veggies, chickpeas, sauerkraut, and quinoa together and mix. Top with pepitas. Drizzle some sauce and add more pepper and salt to your preferred taste (Love and Lemons, 2018).

Stuffed Acorn Squash

This recipe has an earthly flavor from rosemary and sage. There are a lot of variations for this recipe too. The squash halves into natural bowls, which you can roast and serve as a side dish after scooping out the seeds. Apart from that, you can stuff the squash with flavorful fillings, which easily converts it to a main dish!

Ingredients

- Pomegranate arils (a few)
- Parsley
- Chopped rosemary (½ tablespoon)
- Dried cranberries (⅓ cup)
- Apple cider vinegar (1 tablespoon)
- Chopped sage (¼ cup)
- Tamari (1 tablespoon)
- Coarsely chopped walnuts (⅓ cup)
- Minced garlic (3 cloves)
- Chopped yellow onion (½)

- Extra-virgin olive oil (1 tablespoon)
- Tempeh (1 8-ounce package)
- Halved acorn squash (2)
- Diced cremini mushrooms (8 ounces)
- Freshly ground black pepper and sea salt

Steps

1. Use parchment paper to line your baking sheet. Heat the oven to 425°F.
2. Meanwhile, remove seeds from the squash, then put the halves on the baking sheet that you prepared. Drizzle some olive oil on the squash halves and also sprinkle some salt and pepper. With the cut side facing up, roast the squash halves for 40 minutes until they are tender.
3. Cut the tempeh into half-inch cubes while you roast the squash. Put in a steamer basket over a pot with water. Cover the pot, let the water simmer, then steam for 10 minutes. Squeeze out any excess water from the tempeh and crumble it.
4. Put olive oil in a skillet on medium heat. Add black pepper, onion, and half a teaspoon of salt and cook for five minutes. Throw in the mushrooms and cook while stirring for about eight minutes. Stir in the garlic, crumbled tempeh, tamari, walnuts, rosemary, sage, and apple cider vinegar, and then cook for three minutes.
5. As the pan dries, add a quarter cup of water. Put cranberries while stirring and season to taste. Put scoops of filling into the halves of the roasted acorn

squash. Garnish with pomegranates and parsley
(Love and Lemons, 2020).

Rainbow Raw-Maine Taco Boats

Taco boats are appetizing, healthy, delicious, fresh, and easy
to prepare!

Ingredients

- Alfalfa sprouts (½ cup)
- Finely shredded carrots (1 cup)
- Halved cherry tomatoes (1 cup)
- Thinly sliced red cabbage (¾ cup)
- Cubed, medium ripe avocado (1)
- Hemp seeds (1 tablespoon)
- Plain or beet hummus (½ cup)
- Romaine lettuce (1)
- Maple syrup (1 tablespoon)
- Raw, untoasted tahini (⅓ cup)
- Lemon juice (2 tablespoons)
- Water
- Sea salt (1 pinch)

Steps

1. Mix maple syrup, lemon juice, tahini, and salt
   together in a bowl. Whisk these ingredients to
   create a sauce. Form a pourable dressing by adding
   a tablespoon at a time while whisking. Taste, then
   adjust the flavor to your preference.

2. To prepare your 5-minute plain hummus, add undrained chickpeas and garlic cloves in a mixing bowl, then microwave. Combine half chickpea liquid with garlic, chickpeas, tahini, olive oil, salt, and lemon juice in a blender, then process. Keep the other half of chickpea liquid for adding as required when blending. Taste and adjust as you deem fit. With a little, garnish the hummus with some olive oil and paprika.

3. On a serving platter, arrange the lettuce boats. Fill with approximately 30 grams of hummus. You can top with tomatoes, carrots, sprouts, hemp seeds, cabbage, and avocado.

4. Drizzle some tahini sauce and serve! (Minimalist Baker, 2017c)

Vegan BLT Sandwich

This sandwich is fresh, crunchy, smokey, and palatable!

Ingredients

- Thinly sliced medium red or white onion (¼)
- Vegan sandwich bread (2 slices)
- Eggplant bacon (5-6 slices)
- Thinly sliced medium ripe tomato (½)
- Green lettuce (2 leaves)
- Hummus or vegan mayo (2 tablespoons)

Steps

1. Using medium heat, heat the skillet over medium heat. Put the eggplant bacon and cook for two minutes.
2. Toast the bread.
3. Spread hummus or vegan mayo on toasted bread slices to assemble a sandwich. Use onion, tomato, lettuce, and eggplant to top one piece. Cover these toppings with another piece of bread (Minimalist Baker, 2017b).
4. You've got your yummy sandwich!

Vegan Baked Potato

This recipe is satisfying, nourishing, fast, and simple, especially for people with busy schedules. You can bake a lot of potatoes in advance or microwave them right when you need them.

Ingredients

- Salsa (¼ cup)
- Smashed, cubed, or sliced avocado (½)
- Canned black beans (½ cup)
- Large baked potato (1)
- Nutritional yeast (1½ teaspoons)
- Lime wedges
- Cilantro
- Salt and pepper

Steps

1. Preheat the oven to 450°F.
2. Pierce your potato so that steam can escape from it. Microwave it for five minutes or bake for 40 minutes. Check to see if the potato is fully cooked.
3. Slice the potato open and sprinkle nutritional yeast.
4. Add some salsa, avocado, and black beans to the potato. Use salt and pepper to season. Garnish with lime and cilantro (Duclos, 2016). Serve the meal!

Kale Salad With Tahini Dressing

This is one of the lunch recipes that will keep you asking for more. With kale as part of the recipe, there are plenty of nutritional and health benefits. Your gut will also thank you later.

Ingredients

- Hemp seed (3 tablespoons)
- Thinly sliced small radishes (4)
- Ripe avocado (1)
- Mixed greens (6 cups)
- Apple cider vinegar or lemon juice (2 tablespoons)
- Minced garlic (1 clove)
- Shredded red cabbage (1 cup)
- Sweet potato-medium, sliced in ¼ inch rounds (1)
- Zucchini-medium, sliced in ¼ inch rounds (1)
- Water or coconut oil-melted (1 tablespoon)
- Pinch of sea salt (1)
- Curry powder (½ teaspoon)
- Water to thin (¼ cup)

- Coconut aminos (1 tablespoon)
- Garlic powder (½ teaspoon plus more to taste)
- Tahini (⅓ cup)

Steps

1. Heat your oven to 375°F. Arrange cabbage, sweet potatoes, and zucchini on a baking sheet. Drizzle some coconut oil. Also, add sea salt, and curry powder. Toss to mix. Roast in the oven until the sweet potatoes are slightly golden brown and soft. This might take 20 minutes.
2. Prepare quinoa or crispy chickpeas if serving with any of them.
3. To prepare a dressing, add garlic powder, coconut aminos, garlic, and tahini into a bowl. Combine these by whisking. Add some water for thinning until the dressing is pourable. Continue whisking until the dressing is smooth. Taste and adjust seasonings before you set the dressing aside.
4. Add radishes, avocado, hemp seeds, and greens in a huge mixing bowl to prepare a salad. Also, add apple cider vinegar or lemon juice and gently mix.
5. Add the toppings that you prefer: chickpeas, quinoa, and/or roasted veggies. Serve together with the dressing (Minimalist Baker, 2018).

Danny Trejo's Mushroom Asada Tacos

This meal is adapted from the Trejo's Tacos meaty mushrooms that are topped with pumpkin vegan tacos and marinated in asada sauce.

Ingredients

- Orange juice (6 tablespoons)
- Soy sauce (2 tablespoons)
- Lemon juice (½ teaspoon)
- Smoked paprika (1½ teaspoon)
- Garlic cloves (3)
- Cumin-ground (1½ teaspoon)
- Olive oil (6 tablespoons)
- Stemmed and sliced cremini mushrooms (1 pound)
- Salsa verde (¼ cup)
- Quartered limes (3)
- Shredded green cabbage (1½ cup)
- Pepita pesto (½ cup)
- Corn tortillas 6 inches (12)
- Soy sauce (2 tablespoons)
- Cilantro- roughly chopped (¼ cup)
- Orange juice (6 tablespoons)
- Chipotle chile (1)
- Roughly chopped jalapeno (1)

Steps

1. Add orange juice, cilantro, soy sauce, cumin, paprika, white, onion, garlic, adobo sauce, jalapeno,

and lemon in a blender and process. Transfer into a bowl. Add mushrooms to the bowl and toss.

2. Heat the oven to a temperature of 250°F.
3. Add a tablespoon of oil to a skillet and place it over medium heat. Put half of the mushrooms into the pan and sauté for six minutes. Put them in another bowl and set them aside. Do the same with the remaining mushrooms.
4. Place tortillas over a foil paper wrap and put in the oven for 15 minutes.
5. Mix salsa verde and cabbage in another bowl.
6. Evenly top the tortillas with the cabbage mixture, mushroom, and pesto (Parade, 2020). Serving with lime wedges is a great idea!

Grilled Vegan Burger

This is one of the heartiest meals to prepare for lunch.

Ingredients

VG special sauce:

- Vegan mayonnaise (½ cup)
- Ketchup (1½ tablespoon)
- Finely chopped pickled jalapeno (2 teaspoons)
- Finely chopped Giardiniera-style relish (1 tablespoon)

Burgers:

- Finely chopped onion (1)

- Sea salt (¼ teaspoon)
- Vegan cheese slices (4)
- Iceberg lettuce leaves (4)
- Large, sliced tomato (1)
- Sesame seed hamburger buns (4)
- Vegan burger patties (4)
- Steak seasoning (2 teaspoons)
- Finely chopped onion (1)

Steps

1. For the VG special sauce, combine all the ingredients in a small bowl. Set them aside until they are ready to be used.
2. In a large pan, heat the oil over medium-high heat before adding onion and salt.
3. For five minutes, sauté the onion until they are golden brown. Remove them from the pan but keep warm.
4. Heat another pan over medium-high heat. Meanwhile, evenly sprinkle steak seasoning on the patties. Add the patties to the pan and cook for two minutes. Do the same on the other side.
5. Top with cheese and cook for another two minutes. Remove from the pan. Pour excess grease and heat. Put the buns in the pan, with the cut side facing down. Toast them until they turn golden. This takes about 45 seconds, on average.
6. Spread the VG Special Sauce on both sides of the bun.
7. On top of each bottom of the bun, add the patty,

sautéed onions, and lettuce (Ashton, 2017). Cover with the top half of the bun and serve!

Lunchbox Black Bean Quinoa Salad

This is one of the easiest and most simple recipes that can be done in a short space of time. For it to be great, make it the night before for the next day!

Ingredients

- Black beans (½ can)
- Chopped cilantro (2 tablespoons)
- Chopped medium tomatoes (1)
- Corn (¼ cup)
- Dry quinoa (½ cup)
- Minced red onion (¼ cup)
- Sea salt (1 pinch)
- Lime juice (2 tablespoons)
- Olive oil (1 tablespoon)
- Lime zest (1 tablespoon)

Steps

1. Add two cups of water to a pot before adding quinoa. Boil the quinoa while it is covered until there's no water. You need 15 minutes for this.
2. Whisk to make the dressing.
3. Combine veggies, cilantro, beans, and onion with the quinoa. Toss gently in the dressing (Cara, 2011).

9

THE RECIPES—DINNER

Dinner is a crucial part of our day-to-day culture. It's a lovely time to get the family together around the dinner table, talk about your day, and create memories. In American households, dinner usually incorporates some sort of meat or chicken, and you might be wondering how you can have the same dinner impact without them. You definitely can! Plant-based dinner recipes are incredibly delicious. Take a look for yourself in his chapter!

Cauliflower Rice Stir-Fry

This recipe creates a healthy and satiating meal. Cauliflower is a rich source of vitamins, minerals, and protein that will nourish your body. You will have your meal on a table in only 30 minutes.

Ingredients

- Cauliflower (1 head)
- Water (5 tablespoons)
- Almond butter, peanut butter, or sunflower butter (2 tablespoons)
- Sesame or coconut oil (2 teaspoons)
- Lime juice (2 tablespoons)
- Minced fresh ginger (1 tablespoon)
- Coconut aminos (7 tablespoons)
- Chili garlic sauce (4 tablespoons)
- Maple syrup (1 tablespoon)
- Green beans (1½ cups)
- Roasted cashews or slivered toasted almonds (¾ cup)
- Lime wedges
- Chili garlic sauce or sriracha
- Fresh cilantro

Steps

1. Start by preparing your cauliflower rice. Wash the cauliflower and cut it using the medium holes of a box grater. Put the grated cauliflower on a clean towel and squeeze out any excess moisture. Sauté the cauliflower with a tablespoon of oil on medium heat. Cover with a lid and allow the cauliflower to steam for about eight minutes. Season to your preference and set aside.
2. To prepare the sauce, mix lime juice, fresh ginger, nut butter, maple syrup, chili garlic sauce, coconut aminos. Adjust the flavors to your preferred taste.
3. Heat a large-enough skillet over medium to low

heat. Add the cauliflower rice together with some water. Cover with a lid and leave the cauliflower to steam for five minutes. Set aside again.

4. Heat another skillet on medium heat. Add green beans and sesame oil to the hot skillet. Also, add a third of coconut aminos for seasoning. Toss to mix and cover to steam for four minutes.

5. Add cabbage, bell pepper, green onions, and the rest of the coconut aminos. Stir thoroughly and sauté for about four minutes. Add cauliflower rice and cashews to this mixture and stir to mix.

6. Add the sauce and cook for three minutes on medium to low heat (Minimalist Baker, 2017).

7. Enjoy!

Kale Salad in Garlic With Crispy Chickpeas

This recipe is excellent in masking the bitterness of kale, making it a delight to consume. The kale in this recipe also makes you feel fuller for longer, a factor that reduces unnecessary food consumption. Besides, you can prepare this dish in less than 40 minutes!

Ingredients

- Kale (1 bundle)
- Grape or avocado seed oil (1½ tablespoon)
- Chickpeas (1 15-ounce can)
- Sea salt (1 pinch)
- Maple syrup (2 tablespoons)
- Tandoori masala spice blend (3 tablespoons)

- Tahini (⅓ cup)
- Lemon juice (¼ cup)
- Garlic (1 head)
- Hot water
- Olive oil (3½ tablespoons)
- Pepper

Steps

1. Heat the oven to a temperature of 375°F while you peel the bigger garlic cloves apart.
2. Transfer chickpeas to a bowl with salt, seasonings, and oils. Toss these ingredients together.
3. Prepare a baking sheet and add the seasoned chickpeas and the garlic cloves to it—Bake for about 17 minutes. The garlic cloves should be brownish by then, so you should remove and set them aside. Bake the chickpeas further for 13 minutes. Take the chickpeas off the oven and allow them to cool.
4. Peel off the skins from the garlic. Add the tahini, olive oil, maple syrup, lemon juice, salt, pepper, and garlic in a bowl and whisk. Set aside.
5. Put kale in a bowl. Add some olive oil and lemon juice (a tablespoon each). Use your hands to massage the kale to reduce the bitterness and soften its texture. Add the dressings as you prefer.
6. Top the salad with chickpeas (Minimalist Baker, 2015).

Black Bean Soup

Considering that this meal does not need any special equipment, it is pretty easy to prepare. Besides, most of the ingredients that you will use are pantry ones. Get ready to enjoy your meal in 20 minutes!

Ingredients

- Canned beans (15 ounces)
- Olive oil (1 tablespoon)
- Bay leaf (1)
- Vegan butter (1 tablespoon)
- Garlic powder (½ teaspoon)
- Chopped red onion (½)
- Salt and pepper (to taste)
- Cumin (1 teaspoon)
- Smoked paprika (2 teaspoons)
- Water (½ cup)

Steps

1. Add olive oil to a pot. Place the pot on a stove at medium heat. Add chopped onions into the heated oil and stir until tender. This will take about six minutes.
2. Add the garlic powder, bay leaf, cumin, smoked paprika, and the pepper, and salt. After stirring and cooking for a minute, add the water and beans.
3. Bring the pot's contents to boil before lowering the heat so that the beans will simmer. Drop some

vegan butter into the pot. Close the pot with a lid and cook for an additional 10 minutes.

4. Take out the bay leaf, serve your soup, and enjoy! (Michell, 2020).

Vegetarian Meatballs

You can prepare these vegetarian meatballs in about 30 minutes. This healthy, plant-based recipe is delicious and nutritious, too.

Ingredients

- Cauliflower florets (3 cups)
- Oat flour (¾ cup)
- Salt (2 teaspoons)
- Brown rice (1 ½ cups)
- Eggs (4) or egg replacer to make vegan
- Cooked quinoa (3 cups)
- Olive oil
- Spices (1 tablespoon)

Steps

1. Boil the cauliflower florets until they are tender. Drain and set aside. Use a microwave to steam the brown rice. Heat your oven to 400°F.
2. Add the quinoa and cauliflower to a food processor and pulse until the mixture is semi-solid. Thoroughly mix the contents of the food processor with other ingredients in a bowl.

3. Heap one tablespoon with the mixed contents and roll them into a ball. Do this until the whole mixture is used up.
4. Generously brush olive oil onto each ball before baking for 20 minutes.
5. This is better served with yummy salads (Lindsay, 2021).

Vegan Burrito Bowl

A recipe like the vegan burrito bowl is best when you don't have much time to prepare your dinner. It's so easy and quick to prepare—seven minutes is all you need! The vegan burrito bowl is made out of nourishing and satiating ingredients, so there won't be a need for midnight snacks.

Ingredients

- Microwavable brown rice (½ cup)
- Drained and rinsed black beans (½ cup)
- Corn (¼ cup)
- Avocado (½)
- Ripe avocado (½)
- Onion powder (½ teaspoon)
- Finely chopped cilantro (2 tablespoons)
- Chopped romaine (2 cups)
- Chopped bell pepper (½ cup)
- Salsa (¼ cup)
- Juiced lime (½)
- Garlic powder (½ teaspoon)
- Salt and pepper (to taste)

Steps

1. Follow the package instructions and cook the brown rice.
2. Place lettuce into a bowl and top it with the black beans, cilantro, bell pepper, corn, half a cup of rice, and lime juice.
3. Add onion powder, avocado, garlic powder, pepper, and salt into a bowl. Mix and mash these ingredients until you attain a smooth mixture.
4. Scoop on your burrito bowl (Emilie, n.d.).

Tofu Kebabs with Eggplant and Zucchini

Here is a protein-rich recipe that can make your dinner awesome. The eggplant also gives you minerals like potassium, folate, and manganese. Zucchini is an excellent source of vitamins A and C, among other nutrients.

Ingredients

- Grated garlic (1 clove)
- Extra virgin olive oil (1 teaspoon)
- Salt (¼ teaspoon)
- Medium eggplant cut into bite-size chunks (3 cups)
- Red wine vinegar (1 tablespoon)
- Greek seasoning (1 teaspoon)
- Extra-firm tofu cut into bite-sized cubes (6 ounces)
- Medium zucchini cut into bite-size half-moons (2 ½ cups)
- Salt (¼ teaspoon)

Steps

1. Whisk Greek seasoning, garlic, salt, vinegar, and oil in a bowl.
2. Add the tofu, zucchini, and eggplant into the same bowl and toss them gently. Meanwhile, heat your grill to medium.
3. Alternate and evenly thread the eggplant and zucchini onto six skewers. Now, thread the tofu onto two skewers.
4. Oil the rack of the grill and add the kebabs. Cook and turn the grill contents every three minutes. The vegetables will need about 10 minutes for them to become tender, while the tofu requires 12 minutes to be browned.
5. Take the vegetables and tofu off the skewers, serve, and enjoy! (Webster, 2018).

Vegan White Bean Shakshuka

Besides being easy to make, the vegan white bean shakshuka is yummy. The ingredients in this recipe will create a great combination of nutrients, from proteins to minerals like calcium and magnesium. Vitamins A, B6, C, and K are embedded in this recipe.

Ingredients

- Extra virgin olive oil (2 tablespoons)
- Minced garlic (3 cloves)
- Diced tomatoes (28 ounces)

- Ground cumin (1 teaspoon)
- Pepper and salt (½ teaspoon)
- Finely chopped yellow onion (1)
- Cannellini beans (15-ounce can)
- De-stemmed and chopped kale (1 head)
- Smoked paprika (2 teaspoons)
- Dried oregano (1 teaspoon)
- Crushed red pepper (1 pinch)
- Chopped fresh parsley
- Vegan cream cheese

Steps

1. Use medium heat to warm olive oil in a skillet. Throw in onions and cook them until they are transparent. Also, throw in the garlic and cook until it is fragrant. Finally, add kale and continue cooking until it wilts down.
2. Add the following to the skillet: tomatoes, red pepper, cumin, smoked paprika, oregano, pepper, and salt. Gently stir until the sauce begins to simmer.
3. Add white beans to the skillet and cook again. Switch off the heat and set it aside.
4. Use cashew ricotta or vegan cream cheese as a topping. Also, sprinkle parsley and pepper.
5. Serve together with toasted bread (Sarah, 2018).

Roasted Vegan Cauliflower Soup with Parsley-Chive Swirl

This vegan soup recipe has a creamy taste. You will get a silkier texture if you puree the soup in a blender. You need about 75 minutes to get this meal to your table.

Ingredients

- Cut cauliflower florets (18 cups)
- Extra virgin oil (1½ cups)
- Ground pepper (1¾ teaspoons)
- Fresh chives (⅔ cup)
- Leeks with white and green parts only (2)
- Kosher salt (1¾ teaspoons)
- White-wine vinegar (5 teaspoons)
- Fresh parsley (2½ cups)
- Low sodium "no chicken" broth (12 cups)

Steps

1. Make sure your oven is heated to 400°F while you coat two baking sheets with cooking spray.
2. Add a half cup of oil and pepper and salt (one and a quarter teaspoon of each) into a bowl. Add leek and cauliflower and toss.
3. Separate the vegetables in half and share them between the two trays that you prepared in (1) above. Roast, making sure you switch the positions of the pans at regular intervals. This should take between

25 and 30 minutes. The vegetables should appear brownish at the bottom.

4. Add chives, parsley, pepper, and salt (½ teaspoon each) to a blender. Pulse many times before adding a cup of oil. Pulse until the mixture is smooth and put it into a bowl.
5. Get the roasted vegetables to add to a pot before you add broth. Put the pot on high heat and let the contents boil. Lower the heat and allow the pot's contents to simmer for 10 minutes.
6. Puree the soup using a blender. Add vinegar while stirring.
7. Add some herb sauce, swirl it on top, and serve (Gunst, n.d.).

Cannellini Bean Veggie Burger

If you don't want to spend too much time in the kitchen, this recipe is among the ones that you should consider. Packed with fiber and plant-based protein, this recipe is good for your gut microbiota. Along with some plant-based toppings like lettuce, mushroom, and red onion, this recipe is highly nutritious.

Ingredients

- Oat flour (5 tablespoons)
- Garlic powder (1 teaspoon)
- Salt (¼ teaspoon)
- Cannellini beans (1 can)
- Oil (1 tablespoon)

- Smoked paprika (1 teaspoon)
- Chia seeds (1 tablespoon)
- Water (3 tablespoons)

Steps

1. Add water and chia seeds into a bowl and mix together. Allow the contents in the bowl to sit for five minutes before you can stir them.
2. Pour the beans into another bowl. Smash them before adding garlic powder, smoked paprika, salt, oat flour, and the prepared chia egg. Thoroughly mix.
3. Roll the burger mixture into a ball and then cut it into four pieces. Create balls with the pieces and then flatten them to assume the shape of patties.
4. Put the patties into a freezer for 20 minutes until they become firm and frozen.
5. Oil a skillet over medium heat. Add the patties cook for five minutes prior to flipping to the other side.
6. Add the toppings that you prefer and serve (Michell, 2019).

Creamy Vegan Garlic Pasta with Roasted Tomatoes

This fool-proof meal will require 30 minutes of your time to prepare it. Moreover, it is surprisingly savory, rich, and surprisingly satiating. It's a great meal that you can enjoy with your vegan colleagues!

Ingredients

- Grape tomatoes (3 cups)
- Olive oil
- Lemon juice (2 tablespoons)
- Sea salt and black pepper (1 pinch each)
- Unbleached all-purpose flour (4 tablespoons)
- Whole wheat pasta (10 ounces)
- Nutritional yeast (3 tablespoons)
- Medium shallots (2)
- Garlic (2 cloves)
- Unsweetened plant-based milk (2½ cups)
- Vegan parmesan cheese (2 tablespoons)

Steps

1. Toss the tomatoes in salt and olive oil while heating the oven to 400°F. Line a baking sheet with parchment paper and place the tomatoes on it, with the cut side facing up. After baking for 20 minutes, set aside.
2. Prepare your pasta according to the instructions on its package.
3. To prepare the sauce, put a skillet on medium to low heat. Add garlic, shallots, and a tablespoon of olive oil. Add black pepper and salt. Stir regularly while cooking for four minutes.
4. Stir in some flour and thoroughly mix. Add the plant-based milk at intervals while whisking. Add another pinch of salt, along with nutritional yeast. Allow the ingredients to simmer for five minutes.
5. Taste and adjust the seasonings to your preference. Vegan parmesan can add some more flavor.

6. Put the sauce in a blender and process until it's smooth and creamy for an extra creamy sauce. Transfer it back to the pan and allow it to simmer on low heat until it thickens just the way you want it.
7. Check if the sauce tastes to your preference. If yes, then add roasted tomatoes and pasta. Stir well.
8. Garnish with fresh basil, vegan parmesan cheese, and black pepper.
9. Serve and enjoy! (Minimalist Baker, 2014).

Grilled Summer Vegetable Salad

In 25 minutes, you will be enjoying this delicious, gluten-free vegan salad.

Ingredients

- Baby zucchini (2 cups)
- Husked corn (2 ears)
- Divided, extra-virgin olive oil (3 tablespoons)
- Quartered bell peppers (2 large)
- Ground pepper (½ teaspoon)
- Red wine vinegar (1 tablespoon)
- Chopped fresh oregano (2 tablespoons)
- Salt (½ teaspoon)

Steps

1. Preheat the grill to medium-high.

2. Put zucchini, peppers, corn, salt, pepper, and two tablespoons of oil in a large bowl.

3. Oil the grill rack and grill the peppers and zucchini for 6 minutes until they become tender, as well as lightly charred. Grill the corn for 8 minutes.

4. Remove the corn kernels from the cobs. Cut the zucchini into two and chop the peppers into about 1-inch pieces. Put the vegetables in a serving dish. Drizzle with oregano, vinegar, and the remaining tablespoon of oil.

Roasted Root Veggies and Greens On Spiced Lentils

Dinner will be ready to serve 2 in 45 minutes. Enjoy this dairy-free, low-calorie, and gluten-free meal.

Ingredients

- For the lentils
- Water (1 ½ cups)
- Garlic powder (1 teaspoon)
- Black beluga lentils (½ cup)
- Ground cumin (½ teaspoon)
- Ground coriander (½ teaspoon)
- Kosher salt (¼ teaspoon)
- Ground allspice (¼ teaspoon)
- Extra-virgin olive oil (1 teaspoon)
- Lemon juice (2 tablespoons)

For the vegetables:

- Crushed garlic (1 clove)
- Extra-virgin olive oil (1 tablespoon)
- Chopped kale (2 cups)
- Roasted root vegetables (1½ cups)
- Ground pepper (1/8 teaspoon)
- Ground coriander (1 teaspoon)
- Tahini (2 tablespoons)
- Kosher salt (pinch)
- Fresh parsley (for garnishing)

Steps

1. For lentils: In a medium pot, put garlic powder, lentils, water, cumin, ½ teaspoon of coriander, as well as ¼ teaspoon of salt, and bring to a boil. Reduce heat while maintaining a simmer. Cover and cook for 25 to 30 minutes until they become tender.
2. Remove the lid and continue simmering for approximately five more minutes to make the liquid slightly reduce. Drain, then stir in a teaspoon of oil and lemon juice.
3. Vegetables: Use medium heat for heating oil in a large skillet. Add garlic and cook for 1 to 2 minutes. Afterward, put in the roasted root vegetables and cook for about 2 to 4 minutes. Put in kale and cook for 2 to 3 minutes, then add pepper, salt, and coriander.
4. With a tahini topping, serve the vegetables over the lentils. If preferred, garnish with parsley (Fountaine, 2017).

Broccoli Tofu Stir Fry

Enjoy this easy-to-make, healthy, and spicy stir fry. The recipe makes four servings.

Ingredients

For the tofu:

- Corn flour (2 tablespoons)
- Extra-firm tofu (400 grams)
- Ground pepper (¼ teaspoon)
- Salt (½ teaspoon)

For the sauce:

- Light soy sauce (¼ cup)
- Vegetable oil (1½ tablespoons)
- Rice vinegar (2 tablespoons)
- Hoisin sauce (2 teaspoons)
- Chili flakes (1 teaspoon)
- Toasted sesame oil (1 tablespoon)
- Water (¼ cup)
- Corn flour (1 tablespoon)

For the stir fry:

- Oil (1 tablespoon)
- Finely chopped garlic clove (4)
- Green onions
- Toasted sesame seeds
- Whole broccoli florets (1)

- Peeled and finely crushed ginger (1 inch)

Steps

1. Dab the tofu with a paper towel to remove any extra moisture. Chop into ½ inch cubes and mix them with salt, pepper, and corn flour.
2. Whisk all ingredients for the sauce before setting it aside.
3. In a non-stick pan, heat oil and spread out the tofu pieces. Cook both sides until golden brown and remove from the pan.
4. In the same pan, heat oil and put in ginger and garlic. Cook for a minute and pour the sauce into the pan. Stir fry for a few minutes on high heat to thicken the sauce before adding the tofu. Toss everything immediately, then turn the flame off. Use green onions and sesame seeds as toppings and serve (Lander, 2019).

Lemon Pesto Penne

In 45 minutes, you can enjoy this 20-minute lemon pesto penne, which is enough to serve 4.

Ingredients

- Pesto (¼ cup)
- Whole wheat penne (8 ounces)
- Vegan feta cheese (¼ cup)
- Baby broccoli (2 cups)

- Oven-roasted tomatoes (1 cup)
- Fresh basil (cut into ribbons)
- Lemon juice (½ of a lemon)

Steps

1. Follow the package directions to cook the penne. Add the broccoli to boiling water and cook for 1 to 2 minutes so that it turns bright green. Drain and put back to the pan that is under medium heat.
2. To the pan with the baby broccoli and pasta, add tomatoes and sauté until fragrant. Put in the lemon juice, pesto, and half of the vegan feta, before tossing to combine well. Remove from heat, then add basil, and sprinkle the remainder of the vegan feta before serving (Lindsay, 2014).

Butternut Squash Veggie Pizza

The butternut squash veggie pizza is a plant-based meal that the entire family will enjoy. It is best served when fresh but can keep well for up to 3 days. This recipe is enough for eight servings.

Ingredients

For the sauce:

- Cubed butternut squash (3 cups)
- Divided olive oil (2 tablespoons)
- Whole garlic, with skins removed (3 cloves)
- Maple syrup (1 tablespoon)

- Black pepper and sea salt (1 pinch)

For the pizza:

- Chopped red onion (½ cup)
- Dried oregano (1 teaspoon)
- Chopped broccoli, with large stem removed (1½ cups)
- Black pepper and sea salt (1 pinch)
- Vegan parmesan cheese (½ cup)
- Store-bought pizza dough (6 ounces)
- Butternut squash sauce (1 cup)

Steps

1. Preheat the oven to 400°F. Put a rack in the middle of the oven.
2. Add the garlic cloves and cubed butternut squash to a baking sheet before drizzling with pinches of pepper and salt, together with half of the olive oil. Combine by tossing.
3. Bake for about 15 to 20 minutes.
4. Transfer the remainder of olive oil, garlic, squash, and maple syrup to a blender. Purée to make a spreadable and creamy consistency. Taste to your preference then set aside.
5. Use medium heat for heating a large skillet before adding broccoli, onion, a teaspoon of oil, oregano, pepper, and salt, then sauté for about 2 to 3 minutes. Ensure to stir frequently. Put aside.
6. Raise the oven heat to 425°F.

7. Evenly roll out the pizza dough and place it onto a parchment-lined circular baking sheet. For your topping, use 1 cup of sauce veggies, together with sprinkles of oregano and vegan parmesan cheese.
8. Transfer to the oven and bake for 13 to 18 minutes.
9. Slice and serve with the remainder of dried oregano and vegan parmesan cheese (Minimalist Baker, 2015).

You see, you can still have the same impact around the dinner table with these diverse recipes. It's perfect for the entire family, and they give just the right nutrients for you, your significant other, or even your kids. You were told you need to get rid of some unhealthy snacks during a plant-based diet, right? However, what do you replace them with? Find out in the next chapter.

10

THE RECIPES—SNACKS

This chapter will give you popular and delicious recipes that you can use for on-the-go snacks. A variety of recipes that allow you to get important plant-based nutrients will be outlined in this chapter. This chapter also gives you precise ingredients measurements that will help you in your meal preparations.

Pecan Energy Bars

Pecan energy bars are nutritious. They contain fiber, protein, monounsaturated fats, flavonoids, and essential minerals such as zinc, manganese, and copper. Additionally, these energy bars are an easy snack that can be consumed on its own or combined with dried fruit. It will take you 10 minutes to prepare for this mealtime and 30 minutes of cooking time.

Ingredients

- Chia seeds (1 tablespoon)
- Medjool dates (15)
- Raw pecan halves (1 cup)
- Gluten-free oats (½ cup)
- Cinnamon (½ teaspoon)
- Kosher salt (¼ teaspoon)
- Vanilla extract (1 teaspoon)

Steps

1. Heat the oven to 200°F.
2. Take out the pits from the dates using your fingers. Pulse the dates in a food processor until they form a rough texture. Afterward, add in the remainder of the ingredients and process for approximately a minute, ensuring that a crumbly dough is formed.
3. Use parchment paper to line a baking sheet, then place the dough at its center. Roll the dough with a rolling pin to make a rectangular shape that measures six by 10.5 inches. With this measurement, you can cut 14 bars that are 1.5 by 3 inches.
4. To make the texture of the bars less sticky and dry, bake the bars for about 30 minutes. Let the bars cool to room temperature. Store them in a refrigerator in a tightly closed container amid sheets of wax paper. The bars will remain good for a month.

Healthy Apple Nachos

Apple nachos are a great snack, and you can also have them for breakfast or a light lunch. Interestingly, in under 5 minutes, adults and kids will be enjoying the healthy apple nachos they love so much. Eight grams of protein can be obtained for every two tablespoons of nut butter that you use in preparing apple nachos. Additionally, apple nachos are naturally vegan, grain-free, gluten-free, and whole-food plant-based.

Ingredients

- Apples (2)
- Natural nut butter (sunflower, peanut, or almond) (¼ to 1/3 cup)
- Chocolate chips (small handful)
- Shredded coconut (small handful)
- Cinnamon (a sprinkle will do)
- Lemon juice (1 tablespoon)

Toppings (optional)

- Raisins or currants
- Hemp hearts
- Cacao nibs
- Pure maple syrup
- Ground cardamom

Steps

Follow these steps to prepare your apples:

1. Wash your apples, core and cut them into slices that are a quarter-inch in size. Remove the core and the upper and lower ends, which may still harbor some

dirt even after washing.

2. Lay the apple slices on a flat surface so that the inside of the apple is facing up.

3. Put the apple slices in a bowl containing lemon juice and toss to coat.

Here is how to prepare the nut butter :

Expose your nut butter to heat so that it gets warm and a little runny. To warm the butter, place it in a silicon bowl and put it on top of a small pot that contains adequate water to be in contact with the nut butter container. Gently heat the water on low heat until the nut butter becomes warm enough to be pourable. You could also warm the butter for about 20 to 30 seconds in a microwave.

For your serving

1. Place the apple slices in an individual layer on the outside edge of your serving plate. Also, place another small layer over the first slices but ensure that they are layered towards the center of the plate.

2. You can drizzle the nut butter in a zig-zag or circular motion according to your preference.

3. Sprinkle cinnamon, almonds, coconut flakes, and chocolate chips as toppings (Julie, 2020).

Hummus and Veggies

This recipe is easy to prepare and is enough to serve four people. The hummus and veggies snack is vegetarian, plant-based, dairy-free, and gluten-free as well. Below are ingredients and the instructions on how to make your own homemade hummus.

Ingredients

- Medium-sized garlic (1 clove)
- Tahini sauce (¼ cup)
- Chickpeas and aquafaba (1 15-ounce can)
- Kosher salt (¾ teaspoon)
- Large lemon (1)
- Fresh cilantro leaves
- Olive oil
- Toasted pine nuts
- Paprika

Steps

1. Extract juice from the lemon and put it aside.
2. Peel the garlic.
3. Drain the aquafaba from the chickpeas can into a measuring cup.
4. Add garlic to the food processor's bowl and process until completely chopped. Afterward, add kosher salt, two tablespoons of aquafaba, tahini, lemon juice, and chickpeas. Puree for about 30 seconds before scraping down the bowl. Taste, if necessary, add about two more tablespoons of aquafaba and puree for up to 2 minutes until you get a creamy consistency. This can be stored in a refrigerator for about 7 to 10 days.

5. If you wish, make the garnish by baking the pine nuts at 350F for approximately 6 to 8 minutes in a single layer on a rimmed baking sheet. Instead of using the oven, you could also use a dry skillet to toast the pine nuts for a few minutes.

6. For the toppings, add some toasted pine nuts, cilantro leaves, a sprinkle of paprika, and a drizzle of olive oil. Serve with pita bread, crackers, or some veggies.

Vegetable Potato Dippers

Vegetable potato dippers are very delicious, highly nutritious, and easy to make. This recipe has a preparation time of 10 minutes and a cook time of 15 minutes. The vegetable potato dippers are budget-friendly and can be enjoyed by both kids and adults.

Ingredients

- Red lentils (¾ cup)
- Garlic cloves (2)
- Chopped red onion (1)
- Medium-sized carrot (1)
- All-purpose flour (5 tablespoons)
- Uncooked medium-sized potatoes (2)
- Regular paprika powder (1 teaspoon)
- Smoked paprika powder (½ teaspoon)
- Salt
- Black pepper, to taste
- Marjoram (1 teaspoon)

For the sriracha mayonnaise

- Tomato paste (1 teaspoon)
- Vegan mayonnaise (3 tablespoons)
- Garlic powder (1 teaspoon)
- Black pepper (to taste)
- Salt
- Sriracha sauce (to taste)
- Smoked paprika powder (½ teaspoon)

Steps

1. Use the instructions on the package of the red lentils to cook them. Peel and grate the carrot and potatoes.
2. Mix the grated vegetables with the onion, garlic, cooked red lentils, spices, and flour. Stir well.
3. In a large pan, heat some oil and put in approximately 1½ heaped tablespoons for each dipper. Use medium heat to cook them in a non-stick pan for three to four minutes on either side or until golden brown. For an oil-free version of the vegetable potato dippers, put them in the oven for approximately 20 minutes.
4. For the sriracha mayonnaise, mix all of the listed ingredients and stir well.
5. Enjoy your dippers with the sriracha mayonnaise and a green salad (Sina, 2020).

Crispy Roasted Chickpeas

The crispy roasted chickpeas snack is another snack that is plant-based, vegan, dairy-free, and delicious at the same time. This snack has preparation and cooking times of 15 and 60 minutes, respectively.

Ingredients

- Chickpeas (2 15-ounce cans)
- Chili powder (1½ teaspoons)
- Olive oil (2 tablespoons)
- Smoked paprika (½ teaspoon)
- Kosher salt (¾ teaspoon)
- Cumin (1 teaspoon)
- Black pepper (1 teaspoon)

Steps

1. Preheat the oven to 375°F.
2. Rinse, drain, and thoroughly shake off any water from the chickpeas. Afterward, put them on a towel and gently pat them to dry. Remove the chickpea skins as much as possible by placing another towel on top and rubbing them with your hands.
3. Use a medium bowl to mix the chili powder, olive oil, smoked paprika, black pepper, cumin, kosher salt, and chickpeas.
4. A parchment-lined baking sheet is necessary for pouring and spreading the chickpeas into a single

layer. Bake the chickpeas for approximately 45 to 60 minutes until they are dry and crispy. Be sure to shake the pan after every 15 minutes. Your chickpeas should not become extremely hard and dark.

5. Allow them to cool before storing them in an airtight container. You can store them in a dry cupboard for a week (Overhiser, 2019).

Guacamole and Chips

This guacamole snack is vegan, gluten-free, dairy-free, and plant-based. The preparation time for guacamole is 15 minutes. For the tortilla chips, the preparation and cook times are 10 and 15 minutes, respectively.

Ingredients

- Guacamole
- Ripe avocados (3)
- Minced Roma tomato (⅓ cup)
- Lightly chopped cilantro leaves (⅓ cup)
- Minced white onion (⅓ cup)
- Kosher salt (½ teaspoon)
- Fresh lime juice (1 tablespoon)
- Crushed jalapeno or serrano pepper
- Chips
- Corn tortillas (for serving)
- Kosher salt (to taste)

Steps

1. Take out the pit from the avocados. Mince the tomatoes and onions. Roughly slice the cilantro.
2. Scoop the flesh from the avocados into a bowl and mash them until they become creamy. Add the remaining ingredients to the avocado cream. Taste, add seasoning, and minced spicy pepper according to your preference.
3. For the tortilla chips, preheat the oven to 350F. Cut the tortillas into wedges and spread them out in one layer.
4. Bake the wedges for six minutes, using a tong to turn them over. Sprinkle some salt and continue baking for an additional six to nine minutes until they are just beginning to attain a brown color. Take the baked wedges out of the oven and allow them to cool.

Crispy Air-Fried Tofu

This is an oil-free snack that you can have for lunch. It is soft on the inside, has a crispy texture outside, and is perfect when it comes to dipping. The cook time for the air-fried tofu is 10 minutes.

Ingredients

- High protein tofu (1 block)
- Black pepper (¼ teaspoon)
- Smoked paprika (2 teaspoons)
- Garlic powder (¼ teaspoon)

- Salt (¼ teaspoon)
- Ketchup or any other desired condiment

Steps

1. Cut the tofu into small cubes, which you should mix with the spices.
2. Cook for 10 to 15 minutes in an air fryer at 400°F.
3. Enjoy your air-fried tofu with dipping sauce.

Refried Bean Dip and Chips

The refried bean dip is gluten-free, plant-based, and dairy-free. You can prepare this meal in 15 minutes.

Ingredients

- Refried beans (2 cans)
- Mild green chilies 1 (4-ounce can)
- Lime juice (1 tablespoon)
- Smoked paprika (1 teaspoon)
- Ground cumin (1 teaspoon)
- Tortilla chips
- Kosher salt (to taste)
- Hot sauce (1 teaspoon)

Salsa Fresca Topping:

- Finely crushed red onion (2 tablespoons)
- Diced ripe tomato (½ cup)
- Lime juice (1 tablespoon)

- Kosher salt (⅛ teaspoon)
- Chopped cilantro (1 tablespoon)
- Jalapeno pepper (1)
- Ground cumin (⅛ teaspoon)

Steps

1. Ensure that the beans are warm before serving.
2. Add in ground cumin, lime juice, green chilies, hot sauce, and paprika. Stir, taste, and add kosher salt if necessary.
3. For the topping, dice the tomato, cut the cilantro, and finely slice the red onion. Mix the red onion, tomato, cilantro, cumin, kosher salt, and lime juice.
4. Serve the dip in a shallow dish. Use the salsa as a topping, together with thinly sliced jalapeno pepper. Serve the refried bean dip with tortilla chips (Keith, 2020).

Baked Kale Chips

The preparation and cook time for baked kale chips are five and 30 minutes, respectively. Two to three servings can be obtained from this recipe.

Ingredients

- Tuscan kale (1 bunch)
- Onion powder (¼ teaspoon)
- Kosher or fine sea salt (⅛ teaspoon)

Steps

1. Preheat your oven to 275°F.
2. Wash and thoroughly dry your kale using a clean dish towel. Remove the kale stems from the leaves and tear them into the preferred chips' sizes. Slightly toss the dinosaur kale with olive oil in a bowl.
3. Use parchment paper to line a baking sheet and put the kale leaves in one layer. Sprinkle some onion powder and salt.
4. Bake for about 35 minutes. By this time, the kale leaves should be crispy. Allow the kale to cool down and enjoy your snack. If there are leftovers, keep them in a sealed container for a day.

Nut Butter Toast

Try the nut butter toast for another healthy snack. To make it even more delicious, there are many other toppings that you can add.

Ingredients

- Bread (1 slice)
- Nut butter (2 tablespoons)
- Maple syrup or local honey (½ teaspoon)
- Sliced strawberries (6)

Optional toppings include:

- Blackberries or blueberries
- Chia seeds
- Chia jams
- Bee pollen
- Shredded coconut
- Chocolate chips or cacao nibs
- Green apples or sliced bananas

Steps

1. Toast a huge slice of artisan bread.
2. After hulling, make thin slices of the strawberries.
3. When the toast is ready, spread almond butter generously. Drizzle the maple syrup and honey on the toast and top with strawberry slices. You can put more toppings to match your preferences.

Healthy Trail Mix Granola Bars

Healthy trail mix granola bars are paleo-friendly and gluten-free. The preparation and cook times are 5 and 35 minutes, respectively. From this recipe, you can obtain 12 servings.

Ingredients

- Nuts (2 cups)
- Pepitas (¼ cup)
- Dried coconut (½ cup)
- Chia seeds (1 tablespoon)
- Dried cranberries
- Vanilla extract (1 teaspoon)

- Sea salt (¼ teaspoon)
- Maple syrup (¼ cup)

Steps

1. Switch your oven to 325F and line a baking pan with parchment paper.
2. Put the seeds, nuts, salt, and dried fruit in a mixing bowl and stir.
3. Mix maple syrup and the vanilla extract in a separate bowl. Pour the mixture on top of the nuts and stir again until the nuts and dried fruits are homogeneously coated.
4. Pour the mixture into the baking pan and spread it into one layer.
5. Bake for about 35 minutes before cooling for one hour in the pan.
6. Once fully cooled, slice into bars (Bryan, 2020).

Easy Edamame

The easy edamame recipe has a cook time of five minutes and a preparation time of 10 minutes. It is excellent for a vegan diet and serves four people.

Ingredients

- Frozen, pound edamame in pods (1)
- Garlic clove (1 small)
- Toasted sesame oil (½ tablespoon)
- Fine sea or kosher salt (¾ teaspoon)

Steps

1. Put water in a huge saucepan and bring to boil. Add a teaspoon of kosher salt and edamame.
2. Boil the edamame for five minutes until it becomes tender and bright green. Drain after that.
3. Put the edamame in a bowl. Add in salt and toasted sesame oil before grating the garlic clove into the bowl. Ensure that everything is coated by gently tossing. Place in a serving bowl and serve while still warm.

Berry Baked Oatmeal Bars

Berry baked oatmeal bars are a great snack. They are great for adults and kids. Let's have a look at the ingredients and cook instructions in this section.

Ingredients

- Rolled old fashioned oats (2 cups)
- Sea salt (½ teaspoon)
- Baking powder (1 teaspoon)
- Honey or maple syrup (¼ cup)
- Cinnamon (1 teaspoon)
- Apple sauce (½ cup)
- Unsweetened plant-based milk (½ cup)
- Coconut oil (melted) (2 teaspoons)
- Ground flaxseed (2 tablespoons)

- Vanilla extract (1 teaspoon)
- Fresh berries (1 cup)

Steps

1. Preheat the oven to 375F.
2. In a large bowl, mix all ingredients, except for the berries. Stir until thoroughly combined, then carefully fold in a cup of the berries.
3. Pour and evenly spread the batter in a square baking pan that is lined with parchment. Top with the remainder of the berries.
4. Bake for 35 minutes until the baked contents can hold their shape.
5. Remove from the oven and cut into six bars.
6. Enjoy your cold or warm berry-baked oatmeal bars and store leftovers in the fridge for a week.

Almond Butter Stuffed Dates

This excellent snack takes 15 minutes to prepare. In addition to being plant-based, it is also healthy and nutritious.

Ingredients

- Medjool dates (24)
- Nut butter (4 ounces)
- Smoked paprika
- Fresh ground black pepper and sea salt
- Pistachios (3 tablespoons)

Steps

1. Create lengthwise slits into the dates using a knife and take out the pits. Fill the dates with almond butter.
2. Use a rolling pin to crush the pistachios.
3. Sea salt, a small sprinkle of black pepper, and smoked paprika are used to top the almond butter stuffed dates. You can sprinkle small amounts of pistachio dust. If you wish, you can add a tiny drizzle of honey.

Vegan Banana Muffins

These muffins are exceptional. In addition to the banana flavor that they add, they are fluffy and moist. The preparation and cook times are 20 and 30 minutes, respectively.

Ingredients

- All-purpose flour (1½ cups plus 2 tablespoons)
- Rolled oats (¾ cup)
- Baking powder (2 teaspoons)
- Ginger (1 teaspoon)
- Baking soda (1 teaspoon)
- Maple syrup (½ cup)
- Kosher salt (½ teaspoon)
- Vanilla extract (1 tablespoon)
- Large bananas (3)
- Refined coconut oil (½ cup) (half should be at room temperature and the other half, melted)

- Cinnamon, divided (1 tablespoon)
- Turbinado or brown sugar (¼ cup)
- Rum (1 tablespoon)

Steps

1. Preheat your oven to 350F. Add 12 muffin cups into a muffin tin.
2. Mix the one and a half cups of flour, cinnamon, ginger, a half cup rolled oats, kosher salt, baking powder, and soda in a medium-sized bowl.
3. Melt a quarter cup of coconut oil with maple syrup. Combine the maple syrup and coconut oil mixture with vanilla, mashed banana, and rum in another bowl. Combine the wet and dry ingredients. Stir to make a smooth batter.
4. In another bowl, add and mix the remaining two tablespoons of flour, a quarter cup rolled oats, one teaspoon cinnamon, a quarter cup of room temperature coconut oil, as well as the turbinado sugar.
5. Use a fork or pastry cutter to chop the coconut oil into the remainder of the ingredients until a crumbly streusel topping is formed.
6. Evenly divide the batter into muffin cups before topping with streusel.
7. Bake for approximately 25 to 30 minutes until golden brown.
8. Let the muffins cool down, and then serve!

Vegan banana muffins? Yes, please! Doesn't that sound delicious? You see, it's not as bland or boring as you thought it would be. There are so many diverse and delicious things that you can do for your snacks! Now that we talked about all the food we could, there might be some questions in your head that you still don't have the answers to. Hopefully, you'll get them answered with some of the Frequently Asked Questions in the next chapter.

11

PLANT-BASED FAQS

There are so many unanswered questions that might be in your head, and they can make you hesitate to engage on the switch to a plant-based diet. This chapter will clarify your questions. The questions that we will address in this chapter are some of the most asked questions about plant-based diets that can help you on your journey towards a healthy lifestyle.

The Questions

Get the answers to some of the most asked questions with regard to a plant-based diet in this section!

Will I Get Enough Proteins on a Plant-Based Diet?

Yes. You can get enough proteins on a plant-based diet if you know what to eat. Some plant-based protein sources have amounts almost the same as those found in animal sources. For instance, just a half-cup of legumes like lentils, peas, and beans have approximately seven grams of protein. This is almost the same amount of proteins that you will get after eating an ounce of poultry, red meat, and/or fish. Other great sources of proteins are almonds, peanuts, flaxseeds, tofu, edamame, and hemp. You will find proteins in variety — Include good plant-based sources of proteins in every meal, and you are good to go!

Why Should I Switch to a Low-Fat, Plant-Based Diet?

Simply put, a plant-based diet is good for your health. Here, your main objectives are to achieve a healthier lifestyle and a healthier gut. By eating plant-based foods, you protect yourself from an array of diseases like diabetes, hypertension, heart diseases, and stroke. The previous chapters in this book will give you clear explanations with regard to how a plant-based diet protects you from these diseases.

Do I Need Supplements?

Yes, supplements are necessary if you want to provide your body with all the necessary nutrients. There are nutrients that you cannot find in most plant-based foods, yet your body needs them. For instance, vitamin B12 is only available in leafy vegetables, almonds, and legumes, so taking supplements for these nutrients is worth the while.

Can I Switch to a Plant-Based Diet While I'm Pregnant?

Yes, you can! The switch will do good for you and your unborn baby with the richness and healthy nature of plant-based diets.

Are Soy Products Healthy?

There are a ton of health benefits that are associated with soy products. Just to mention a few, soy products will help you with your heart and bone health. These products also assist you in dealing with menopausal symptoms. Soy products contain isoflavones that work just like estrogen in reducing hot flashes.

Does a Plant-Based Diet Require a Lot of Planning?

Yes and no. When you begin your transition to a plant-based diet, you might need a lot of planning to help you stick to the diet. However, as time progresses and you have a hang of the diet, it becomes part of your lifestyle. At this point, planning will become relatively easier.

How Much Should I Eat in a Plant-Based Diet?

There are limitations on how much you should eat when you are on a plant-based diet. Eat until you're satiated. In fact, there is no need to be counting calories because plant-based diets are relatively healthy.

Is a Plant-Based Diet Expensive?

Not at all! Grains, nuts, seeds, and plants are among the least expensive foods around. Therefore, plant-based foods are quite affordable.

What are the Good Sources of Plant-Based Protein?

Plant-based foods contain a great deal of proteins. Some of the best sources of proteins are tofu, chia seeds, quinoa, nut butters, oats, broccoli, and lentils. Please note that nearly every plant-based food you consume does have some proteins.

There you have it! All the information you may need is right here at your fingertips. You must feel more confident in making the transition, and I'll be there to help you through the entire process.

CONCLUSION

Taking care of your gut is one of the major responsibilities that you need to take care of. One of the easiest ways to do so is through knowing what to eat. In this book, we recommend that you eat a plant-based diet, not only for the health of your gut but for your overall health, too. Plant-based diets have nutrients that nourish microorganisms that stay in your gut. This can either increase the numbers of some microbial strains or even widen the diversity of the gut microbiota.

There are various reasons why you should take care of your gut. This is where all the digestion and absorption of nutrients take place. Your mood and other emotions that are controlled by serotonin are predominantly controlled in the gut. This is because most of this hormone is released in the gut. Your gastrointestinal tract regulates a remarkable part of your immune system.

Eating a plant-based diet will also benefit the rest of your body, other than the gut. The risks of some diseases like heart disease, diabetes, high blood pressure, stroke, and some cancers are significantly reduced. A plant-based diet can contribute to intelligence, even emotionally. Moreover, plant-based diets do not only benefit you; it also encourages kindness toward animals and the environment. The wastes that are produced in processing animal products are more than those released when dealing with plant-based products. More importantly, a plant-based lifestyle is less expensive and affordable.

Moving to a plant-based diet might not be so easy, but it is worth the while. Many other people might be going through the same struggles that you are facing in making the transition work. Some faced them already, and conquered—I am one of those. If I could do it, trust me, you also can. Just try to make the transition as gradual as possible so that it becomes more enjoyable.

Take the initiative and take care of your gut by transitioning to a plant-based diet. If you have enjoyed his book and you want it to reach out to even more people, kindly leave a positive review. All the best in taking good care of your gut!

LEAVE A 1-CLICK REVIEW

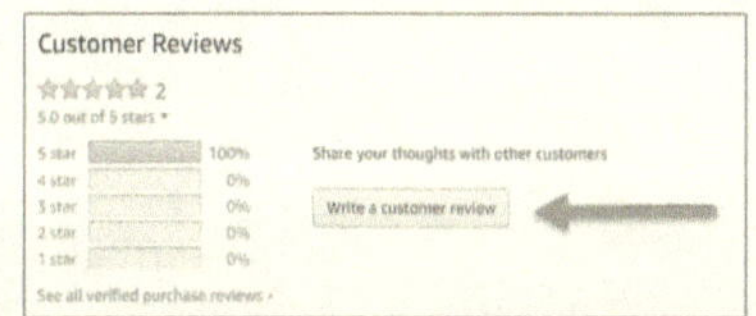

I would be incredibly <u>thankful</u> if you could take just 60 seconds to write a brief review on Amazon, even if its just a few sentences!

OTHER BOOKS YOU'LL LOVE

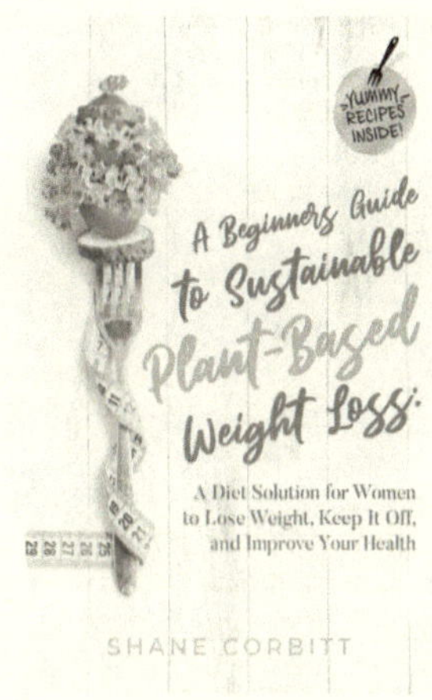

Book Link

FREE PLANT-BASED COOKBOOK

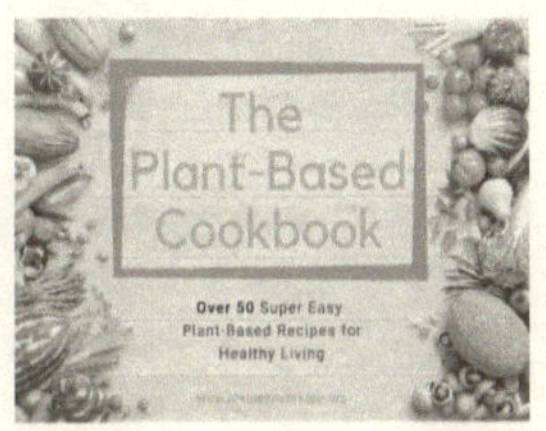

A Free Gift to My Readers
Over 50 Plant-Based Recipes. Download and Start Eating
Healthy Today!
www.createyourhappy.org/cookbook

REFERENCES

4 fast facts about the gut-brain connection. (n.d.). NCCIH. https://www.nccih.nih.gov/news/events/4-fast-facts-about-the-gutbrain-connection

Akbaraly, T. N., Brunner, E. J., Ferrie, J. E., Marmot, M. G., Kivimaki, M., & Singh-Manoux, A. (2009). Dietary pattern and depressive symptoms in middle age. *British Journal of Psychiatry, 195*(5), 408–413. https://doi.org/10.1192/bjp.bp.108.058925

Ashton, A. (2017, May 26). *Veggie grill vegan all-american burger*. Parade: Entertainment, Recipes, Health, Life, Holidays. https://parade.com/842230/alisonashton/veggie-grill-vegan-all-american-burger/

Bamberger, C., Rossmeier, A., Lechner, K., Wu, L., Waldmann, E., Fischer, S., Stark, R. G., Altenhofer, J., Henze, K., & Parhofer, K. G. (2018). A walnut-enriched diet affects gut microbiome in healthy caucasian subjects: A randomized, controlled trial. *Nutrients, 10*(2). https://doi.org/10.3390/nu10020244

Bancos, I. (2018, December). *Serotonin.* www.hormone.org. https://www.hormone.org/your-health-and-hormones/ glands-and-hormones-a-to-z/hormones/serotonin

BBC Radio 4. (2018, October 9). *10 smart facts about your gut.* www.mentalfloss.com. https://www.mentalfloss.com/article/ 64685/10-brainy-facts-about-your-gut-its-smarter-you-think

Bonsall, A. (n.d.). *The digestive system.* Patient.info. https:// patient.info/news-and-features/the-digestive-system

Cara. (2011, August 26). *Lunchbox black bean quinoa salad.* Fork and Beans. http://www.forkandbeans.com/2011/08/26/ lunchbox-black-bean-quinoa-salad/

Carpenter, S. (2021). *That gut feeling.* Apa.org. https://www. apa.org/monitor/2012/09/gut-feeling

Choi, Y., Larson, N., Steffen, L. M., Schreiner, P. J., Gallaher, D. D., Duprez, D. A., Shikany, J. M., Rana, J. S., & Jacobs, D. R. (2021). Plant-centered diet and risk of incident cardiovascular disease during young to middle adulthood. *Journal of the American Heart Association, 10*(16). https://doi.org/10.1161/ jaha.120.020718

Christian, C. (2018, December 26). *Creamy wild rice soup.* Forks over Knives. https://www.forksoverknives.com/recipes/ vegan-soups-stews/creamy-wild-rice-soup/

Chuang, S.-Y., Chiu, T. H. T., Lee, C.-Y., Liu, T.-T., Tsao, C. K., Hsiung, C. A., & Chiu, Y.-F. (2016a). Vegetarian diet reduces the risk of hypertension independent of abdominal obesity and inflammation: A prospective study. *Journal of Hypertension,* 34(11), 2164–2171. https://doi.org/10. 1097/HJH.0000000000001068

Chuang, S.-Y., Chiu, T. H. T., Lee, C.-Y., Liu, T.-T., Tsao, C. K., Hsiung, C. A., & Chiu, Y.-F. (2016b). Vegetarian diet reduces the risk of hypertension independent of abdominal obesity and inflammation: a prospective study. *Journal of Hypertension,* 34(11), 2164–2171. https://doi.org/10. 1097/HJH.0000000000001068

Cleveland Clinic. (n.d.). *Structure and function of the digestive system: How it works.* Cleveland Clinic. https://my. clevelandclinic.org/health/articles/7041-the-structure-and-function-of-the-digestive-system

Collado, M. C., Engen, P. A., Bandín, C., Cabrera-Rubio, R., Voigt, R. M., Green, S. J., Naqib, A., Keshavarzian, A., Scheer, F. A. J. L., & Garaulet, M. (2018). Timing of food intake impacts daily rhythms of human salivary microbiota: a randomized, crossover study. *The FASEB Journal,* 32(4), 2060–2072. https://doi.org/10.1096/fj.201700697rr

Crawford, N. (2011, May 7). *How unhealthy foods affect the body.* livestrong.com. https://www.livestrong.com/article/436610-how-unhealthy-foods-affect-the-body/

Danone Nutricia Research. (n.d.). *The central role of the gut.* Danone Nutricia Research. https://www.nutriciaresearch. com/gut-and-microbiology/the-central-role-of-the-gut/

David, L. A., Materna, A. C., Friedman, J., Baptista, M. I. C., Blackburn, M. C., Perrotta, A., Erdman, S. E., & Alm, E. J.

(2016). Erratum to: Host lifestyle affects human microbiota on daily timescales. *Genome Biology, 17*(1). https://doi.org/10.1186/s13059-016-0988-y

David, L. A., Maurice, C. F., Carmody, R. N., Gootenberg, D. B., Button, J. E., Wolfe, B. E., Ling, A. V., Devlin, A. S., Varma, Y., Fischbach, M. A., Biddinger, S. B., Dutton, R. J., & Turnbaugh, P. J. (2013). Diet rapidly and reproducibly alters the human gut microbiome. *Nature, 505*(7484), 559–563. https://doi.org/10.1038/nature12820

De Filippis, F., Pellegrini, N., Vannini, L., Jeffery, I. B., La Storia, A., Laghi, L., Serrazanetti, D. I., Di Cagno, R., Ferrocino, I., Lazzi, C., Turroni, S., Cocolin, L., Brigidi, P., Neviani, E., Gobbetti, M., O'Toole, P. W., & Ercolini, D. (2015). High-level adherence to a Mediterranean diet beneficially impacts the gut microbiota and associated metabolome. *Gut, 65*(11), 1812–1821. https://doi.org/10.1136/gutjnl-2015-309957

Debret, C. (2021, October 19). *The dangers of low cholesterol and nutrient deficiency on a plant-based diet*. One Green Planet. https://www.onegreenplanet.org/natural-health/dangers-low-cholesterol-nutrient-deficiency-plant-based-diet/

Digestive, C. (2021, June 22). *The signs and symptoms of an unhealthy gut*. Carolina Digestive. https://carolinadigestive.com/about-us/news/the-signs-and-symptoms-of-an-unhealthy-gut

Dix, M. (2020, August 25). *7 signs of an unhealthy gut and 7 ways to improve gut health*. Healthline. https://www.healthline.com/health/gut-health

Donahue, A. (n.d.). *Overnight chia seed pudding (plant-based).*

MamaSezz. https://www.mamasezz.com/blogs/recipes/overnight-chia-seed-pudding-plant-based

Duclos, A. (2016, July 11). *"Nacho" vegan baked potato recipe*. Forks over Knives. https://www.forksoverknives.com/recipes/vegan-baked-stuffed/nacho-baked-potato/

Eat the 80. (n.d.). *Love your gut: Why a healthy gut is so important*. www.eatthe80.com. https://www.eatthe80.com/love-your-gut-why-a-healthy-gut-is-so-important/

Emilie. (n.d.). *Vegan burrito bowl recipe*. www.yummly.com. https://www.yummly.com/recipe/Vegan-Burrito-Bowl-2252304

Ercolini, D., & Fogliano, V. (2018). Food design to feed the human gut microbiota. *Journal of Agricultural and Food Chemistry, 66*(15), 3754–3758. https://doi.org/10.1021/acs.jafc.8b00456

Esophagus: Anatomy, function and conditions. (n.d.). Cleveland Clinic. https://my.clevelandclinic.org/health/body/21728-esophagus

Fawley, C. D. (n.d.-a). *Plant-based breakfast recipe for oatmeal muffins*. MamaSezz. Retrieved December 22, 2021, from https://www.mamasezz.com/blogs/recipes/plant-based-breakfast-oatmeal-muffins

Fawley, C. D. (n.d.-b). *Plant-based breakfast recipe: Chipotle black bean avocado toast*. MamaSezz. https://www.mamasezz.com/blogs/recipes/plant-based-breakfast-recipe-chipotle-black-bean-avocado-toast

Ferdowsian, H. R., & Barnard, N. D. (2009). Effects of plant-based diets on plasma lipids. *The American Journal of Cardiology, 104*(7), 947–956. https://doi.org/10.1016/j.amjcard.2009.05.032

Fields, H. (2014). *The gut: Where bacteria and the immune system meet.* Hopkinsmedicine.org. https://www.hopkinsmedicine.org/research/advancements-in-research/fundamentals/in-depth/the-gut-where-bacteria-and-immune-system-meet

Forks and Knives. (2015, August 31). *Vegan omelette recipe made with chickpea.* Forks over Knives. https://www.forksoverknives.com/recipes/vegan-breakfast/chickpea-omelet/

Forks Over Knives. (2017, January 23). *Orange French toast.* Forks over Knives. https://www.forksoverknives.com/recipes/vegan-breakfast/orange-french-toast/

Forks Over Knives. (2018, August 15). *Tex-Mex pita pizzas.* Forks over Knives. https://www.forksoverknives.com/recipes/vegan-baked-stuffed/tex-mex-pita-pizzas/

Glick-Bauer, M., & Yeh, M.-C. (2014). The health advantage of a vegan diet: Exploring the gut microbiota connection. *Nutrients, 6*(11), 4822–4838. https://doi.org/10.3390/nu6114822

Gregor, M. (2007, September 26). *IQ of vegetarian children.* Nutritionfacts.org. https://nutritionfacts.org/video/iq-of-vegetarian-children-2/

Gunst, K. (n.d.). *Roasted vegan cauliflower soup with parsley-chive swirl.* EatingWell. https://www.eatingwell.com/recipe/

262133/roasted-vegan-cauliflower-soup-with-parsley-chive-swirl/

Heartburn and acid reflux: What you need to know. (n.d.). Cedars-Sinai. https://www.cedars-sinai.org/blog/what-causes-heartburn-and-acid-reflux.html

Hentges, D. J., Maier, B. R., Burton, G. C., Flynn, M. A., & Tsutakawa, R. K. (1977). Effect of a high-beef diet on the fecal bacterial flora of humans. *Cancer Research, 37*(2), 568–571. https://pubmed.ncbi.nlm.nih.gov/832279/

How dietary fibre cuts your cancer risk. (n.d.). www.cancer-sa.org.au. https://www.cancersa.org.au/prevention/lifestyle-factors/diet/how-dietary-fibre-cuts-your-cancer-risk/

Hu, D., Huang, J., Wang, Y., Zhang, D., & Qu, Y. (2014). Fruits and vegetables consumption and risk of stroke: a meta-analysis of prospective cohort studies. *Stroke, 45*(6), 1613–1619. https://doi.org/10.1161/STROKEAHA.114.004836

Huzar, T. (2021, April 3). *Boosting fiber intake for 2 weeks alters the microbiome.* www.medicalnewstoday.com. https://www.medicalnewstoday.com/articles/short-term-increase-in-fiber-alters-gut-microbiome

Johns Hopkins Medicine. (2019). *The brain-gut connection.* John Hopkins Medicine. https://www.hopkinsmedicine.org/health/wellness-and-prevention/the-brain-gut-connection

Johnson, A. J., Vangay, P., Al-Ghalith, G. A., Hillmann, B. M., Ward, T. L., Shields-Cutler, R. R., Kim, A. D., Shmagel, A. K., Syed, A. N., Walter, J., Menon, R., Koecher, K., & Knights, D. (2019). Daily sampling reveals personalized diet-microbiome associations in humans. *Cell Host & Microbe*, 25(6), 789-802.e5. https://doi.org/10.1016/j.chom.2019.05.005

Karlsen, M. (2017, January 5). *Apple-lemon breakfast bowl.* Forks over Knives. https://www.forksoverknives.com/recipes/vegan-breakfast/apple-lemon-breakfast/

Keim, N. L., & Martin, R. J. (2014). Dietary whole grain–microbiota interactions: Insights into mechanisms for human health. *Advances in Nutrition*, 5(5), 556–557. https://doi.org/10.3945/an.114.006536

Kim, C. H., Park, J., & Kim, M. (2014). Gut microbiota-derived short-chain fatty acids, t cells, and inflammation. *Immune Network*, 14(6), 277. https://doi.org/10.4110/in.2014.14.6.277

Kim, H., Caulfield, L. E., Garcia-Larsen, V., Steffen, L. M., Coresh, J., & Rebholz, C. M. (2019). Plant-based diets are associated with a lower risk of incident cardiovascular disease, cardiovascular disease mortality, and all-cause mortality in a general population of middle-aged adults. *Journal of the American Heart Association*, 8(16). https://doi.org/10.1161/jaha.119.012865

Klimenko, N., Tyakht, A., Popenko, A., Vasiliev, A., Altukhov, I., Ischenko, D., Shashkova, T., Efimova, D., Nikogosov, D., Osipenko, D., Musienko, S., Selezneva, K., Baranova, A., Kurilshikov, A., Toshchakov, S., Korzhenkov, A., Samarov, N., Shevchenko, M., Tepliuk, A., & Alexeev, D. (2018). Microbiome responses to an uncontrolled short-term diet intervention in the Frame of the Citizen Science Project. *Nutrients*, 10(5), 576. https://doi.org/10.3390/nu10050576

Lanou, A. J., & Svenson, B. (2010). Reduced cancer risk in

vegetarians: An analysis of recent reports. *Cancer Management and Research*, 1. https://doi.org/10.2147/cmr.s6910

Lashner, B. (2016, March 29). *9 amazing, weird facts about your gut*. Health Essentials from Cleveland Clinic. https://health.clevelandclinic.org/9-amazing-weird-facts-gut/

Leeming, E. R., Johnson, A. J., Spector, T. D., & Le Roy, C. I. (2019). Effect of diet on the gut microbiota: Rethinking intervention duration. *Nutrients*, *11*(12), 2862. https://doi.org/10.3390/nu11122862

Levine, Morgan E., Suarez, Jorge A., Brandhorst, S., Balasubramanian, P., Cheng, C.-W., Madia, F., Fontana, L., Mirisola, Mario G., Guevara-Aguirre, J., Wan, J., Passarino, G., Kennedy, Brian K., Wei, M., Cohen, P., Crimmins, Eileen M., & Longo, Valter D. (2014). Low protein intake is associated with a major reduction in igf-1, cancer, and overall mortality in the 65 and younger but not older population. *Cell Metabolism*, *19*(3), 407–417. https://doi.org/10.1016/j.cmet.2014.02.006

Lindsay. (2021, September 3). *30 minute vegetarian meatballs*. Pinch of Yum. https://pinchofyum.com/30-minute-vegetarian-meatballs?utm_campaign=yummly&utm_medium=yummly&utm_source=yummly

Link, R. (2021, November 5). *Top 10 foods highest in calories to avoid for weight loss*. Myfooddata. https://www.myfooddata.com/articles/high-calorie-foods-to-avoid.php

Link-Amster, H., Rochat, F., Saudan, K. Y., Mignot, O., & Aeschlimann, J. M. (1994). Modulation of a specific humoral immune response and changes in intestinal flora mediated through fermented milk intake. *FEMS Immunology and Medical Microbiology*, *10*(1), 55–63. https://doi.org/10.1111/j.1574-695X.1994.tb00011.x

Liz. (2018, March 8). *Chickpea salad sandwich*. I Heart Vegetables. https://iheartvegetables.com/green-goddess-chickpea-sandwiches/

Love and Lemons. (2017, March 28). *Best Buddha bowl*. Love and Lemons. https://www.loveandlemons.com/buddha-bowl-recipe/

Love and Lemons. (2018, April 3). *Roasted veggie grain bowl*. Love and Lemons. https://www.loveandlemons.com/grain-bowl/

Love and Lemons. (2020, November 15). *Stuffed acorn squash*. Love and Lemons. https://www.loveandlemons.com/stuffed-acorn-squash/

Macey, D. (2017, December 14). *How to transition to a plant-based diet*. Running on Real Food. https://runningonrealfood.com/how-to-transition-to-a-plant-based-diet/

Masrul, M., & Nindrea, R. D. (2019). Dietary fibre protective against colorectal cancer patients in asia: a meta-analysis. *Open Access Macedonian Journal of Medical Sciences*, *7*(10), 1723–1727. https://doi.org/10.3889/oamjms.2019.265

Matijašić, B. B., Obermajer, T., Lipoglavšek, L., Grabnar, I., Avguštin, G., & Rogelj, I. (2013). Association of dietary type with fecal microbiota in vegetarians and omnivores in Slovenia. *European Journal of Nutrition*, *53*(4), 1051–1064. https://doi.org/10.1007/s00394-013-0607-6

Mayfair. (2019). *How does the gastrointestinal system change with age?* https://www.radiology.ca/article/how-does-gastrointestinal-system-change-age

McDougall, H. (2014, May 21). *Lentil vegetable soup recipe.* Forks over Knives. https://www.forksoverknives.com/recipes/vegan-soups-stews/lentil-vegetable-soup/

MedlinePlus. (2013). *Stomach acid test: MedlinePlus Medical Encyclopedia.* Medlineplus.gov. https://medlineplus.gov/ency/article/003883.htm

Michell, A. (2019, February 22). *Cannellini bean veggie burgers.* Plant Based and Broke: Cheap and Easy Plant-Based Recipes. https://plantbasedandbroke.com/easy-plant-based-veggie-burgers-with-cannellini-beans/

Michell, A. (2020, August 10). *20-minute black bean soup.* Plant Based and Broke: Cheap and Easy Plant-Based Recipes. https://plantbasedandbroke.com/20-minute-black-bean-soup/

Migala, J. (2020, May 1). *6 expert tips for switching to a plant-based diet.* EverydayHealth.com. https://www.everydayhealth.com/diet-nutrition/switching-to-a-more-plant-based-diet-tips-for-making-it-happen/

Minimalist Baker. (2015, April 9). *Garlicky kale salad with crispy chickpeas.* Minimalist Baker. https://minimalistbaker.com/garlicky-kale-salad-with-crispy-chickpeas/

Minimalist Baker. (2017a, January 2). *Collard green spring rolls plus sunflower butter dipping sauce.* Minimalist Baker. https://

minimalistbaker.com/collard-green-spring-rolls-sunbutter-dipping-sauce/

Minimalist Baker. (2017b, March 8). *Vegan "BLT" sandwich.* Minimalist Baker. https://minimalistbaker.com/vegan-blt-sandwich/

Minimalist Baker. (2017c, July 3). *Rainbow "Raw-maine" taco boats.* Minimalist Baker. https://minimalistbaker.com/rainbow-raw-maine-taco-boats/

Minimalist Baker. (2017d, November 3). *30-minute cauliflower rice stir-fry.* Minimalist Baker. https://minimalistbaker.com/30-minute-cauliflower-rice-stir-fry/

Minimalist Baker. (2018, February 22). *Abundant kale salad with savory tahini dressing.* Minimalist Baker. https://minimalistbaker.com/abundance-kale-salad-with-savory-tahini-dressing/

Morris, M. C., Wang, Y., Barnes, L. L., Bennett, D. A., Dawson-Hughes, B., & Booth, S. L. (2017). Nutrients and bioactives in green leafy vegetables and cognitive decline. *Neurology, 90*(3), e214–e222. https://doi.org/10.1212/wnl.0000000000004815

Nall, R. (2018, September 5). *Chemical digestion: Definition, purpose, starting point, and more.* Healthline. https://www.healthline.com/health/chemical-digestion

National Institutes of Health. (2013). *Energy balance and obesity, healthy weight basics. NIH.* https://www.nhlbi.nih.gov/health/educational/wecan/healthy-weight-basics/balance.htm

Nazish, N. (2018, November 30). *How to smoothly transition to a plant-based diet.* Forbes. https://www.forbes.com/sites/nomanazish/2018/11/30/how-to-smoothly-transition-to-a-plant-based-diet/?sh=165dd1450dcb

Overhiser, S. (2017, July 30). *Maple Pecan Homemade Muesli.* A Couple Cooks. https://www.acouplecooks.com/cinnamon-pecan-homemade-breakfast-cereal/

Overhiser, S. (2018, January 9). *Vegan French toast with caramelized bananas.* A Couple Cooks. https://www.acouple-cooks.com/vegan-banana-french-toast/

Overhiser, S. (2020, September 28). *Banana baked oatmeal.* A Couple Cooks. https://www.acouplecooks.com/banana-baked-oatmeal/

Parade. (2020, March 20). *Danny Trejo's vegan mushroom tacos will blow your mind.* Parade: Entertainment, Recipes, Health, Life, Holidays. https://parade.com/991086/parade/danny-trejos-vegan-mushroom-tacos-will-blow-your-mind/

Physicians Committee for Responsible Medicine. (n.d.). *A vegan diet: Eating for the environment.* Physicians Committee for Responsible Medicine. https://www.pcrm.org/good-nutrition/vegan-diet-environment

Physicians Committee for Responsible Medicine. (2019). *Alzheimer's Disease.* Physicians Committee for Responsible Medicine. https://www.pcrm.org/health-topics/alzheimers

Plant Based News. (2019, June 26). *Thinking of quitting your vegan diet? Doctors address 5 common health questions.* Plant

Based News. https://plantbasednews.org/lifestyle/quitting-vegan-diet-doctors-5-common-health-questions/

Rajkumar, H., Mahmood, N., Kumar, M., Varikuti, S. R., Challa, H. R., & Myakala, S. P. (2014). Effect of probiotic (VSL#3) and omega-3 on lipid profile, insulin sensitivity, inflammatory markers, and gut colonization in overweight adults: a randomized, controlled trial. *Mediators of Inflammation, 2014*, 1–8. https://doi.org/10.1155/2014/348959

Rosenfeld, J. (2018, October 9). *10 smart facts about your gut.* www.mentalfloss.com. https://www.mentalfloss.com/article/64685/10-brainy-facts-about-your-gut-its-smarter-you-think

Rosewell Park. (2019, December 23). *For the health benefits of phytochemicals, "Eat a rainbow."* Roswell Park Comprehensive Cancer Center. https://www.roswellpark.org/cancertalk/201912/health-benefits-phytochemicals-eat-rainbow

Saito, Y. A., Schoenfeld, P., & Locke, G. R. (2002). The epidemiology of irritable bowel syndrome in North America: a systematic review. *The American Journal of Gastroenterology, 97*(8), 1910–1915. https://doi.org/10.1111/j.1572-0241.2002.05913.x

Sarah. (2018, September 17). *One-pot vegan white bean shakshuka recipe.* www.yummly.com. https://www.yummly.com/recipe/One-Pot-Vegan-White-Bean-Shakshuka-2642479

Secretion of bile and the role of bile acids in digestion. (n.d.). www.vivo.colostate.edu. http://www.vivo.colostate.edu/hbooks/pathphys/digestion/liver/bile.html

Shen, J., Zuo, Z.-X., & Mao, A.-P. (2014). Effect of probiotics on inducing remission and maintaining therapy in ulcerative colitis, Crohn's disease, and pouchitis: meta-analysis of randomized controlled trials. *Inflammatory Bowel Diseases, 20*(1), 21–35. https://doi.org/10.1097/01.MIB.0000437495.30052.be

Shmerling, R. H. (2018, August 22). *Autoimmune disease and stress: Is there a link? - Harvard Health Blog.* Harvard Health Blog. https://www.health.harvard.edu/blog/autoimmune-disease-and-stress-is-there-a-link-2018071114230

Singh, R. K., Chang, H.-W., Yan, D., Lee, K. M., Ucmak, D., Wong, K., Abrouk, M., Farahnik, B., Nakamura, M., Zhu, T. H., Bhutani, T., & Liao, W. (2017). Influence of diet on the gut microbiome and implications for human health. *Journal of Translational Medicine, 15*(1). https://doi.org/10.1186/s12967-017-1175-y

So, D., Whelan, K., Rossi, M., Morrison, M., Holtmann, G., Kelly, J. T., Shanahan, E. R., Staudacher, H. M., & Campbell, K. L. (2018). Dietary fiber intervention on gut microbiota composition in healthy adults: A systematic review and meta-analysis. *The American Journal of Clinical Nutrition, 107*(6), 965–983. https://doi.org/10.1093/ajcn/nqy041

Splendid Spoon. (2020, February 12). *IQ of vegetarian children.* Nutritionfacts.org. https://nutritionfacts.org/video/iq-of-vegetarian-children-2/

Sroufe, D. (2015a, August 20). *Plant-based granola with banana and almond.* Forks over Knives. https://www.forksoverknives.com/recipes/vegan-breakfast/banana-almond-vegan-granola-recipe/

Sroufe, D. (2015b, October 16). *Polenta with pears and cranber-*

ries: Plant-based vegan recipe.* Forks over Knives. https://www.forksoverknives.com/recipes/vegan-breakfast/vegan-polenta-pears-cranberries/

Sroufe, D. (2016, January 20). *Egyptian breakfast beans (ful medames).* Forks over Knives. https://www.forksoverknives.com/recipes/vegan-breakfast/egyptian-breakfast-beans-ful-medames/

Sroufe, D. (2018, September 5). *Healthy oatmeal recipe with fruits and nuts.* Forks over Knives. https://www.forksoverknives.com/recipes/vegan-breakfast/fruit-and-nut-healthy-oatmeal/

Sung, H., Ferlay, J., Siegel, R. L., Laversanne, M., Soerjomataram, I., Jemal, A., & Bray, F. (2021). Global cancer statistics 2020: GLOBOCAN estimates of incidence and mortality worldwide for 36 cancers in 185 countries. *CA: A Cancer Journal for Clinicians, 71*(3), 209–249. https://doi.org/10.3322/caac.21660

Syn, M. (2021, October 11). *What Is a plant-based diet?* Verywell Fit. https://www.verywellfit.com/plant-based-diet-recipes-tips-guidelines-4174728

Thacker, D. (2021, September 8). *Gluten-free chocolate chip pancakes.* Forks over Knives. https://www.forksoverknives.com/recipes/vegan-breakfast/gluten-free-chocolate-chip-pancakes/

Thaiss, Christoph A., Zeevi, D., Levy, M., Zilberman-Schapira, G., Suez, J., Tengeler, Anouk C., Abramson, L., Katz, Meirav N., Korem, T., Zmora, N., Kuperman, Y., Biton, I., Gilad, S., Harmelin, A., Shapiro, H., Halpern, Z., Segal, E.,

& Elinav, E. (2014). Transkingdom control of microbiota diurnal oscillations promotes metabolic homeostasis. *Cell, 159*(3), 514–529. https://doi.org/10.1016/j.cell.2014.09.048

Tomova, A., Bukovsky, I., Rembert, E., Yonas, W., Alwarith, J., Barnard, N. D., & Kahleova, H. (2019). The effects of vegetarian and vegan diets on gut microbiota. *Frontiers in Nutrition, 6*(47). https://doi.org/10.3389/fnut.2019.00047

Towery, P., Guffey, J. S., Doerflein, C., Stroup, K., Saucedo, S., & Taylor, J. (2018). Chronic musculoskeletal pain and function improve with a plant-based diet. *Complementary Therapies in Medicine, 40*, 64–69. https://doi.org/10.1016/j.ctim.2018.08.001

Turner-McGrievy, G. M., Davidson, C. R., Wingard, E. E., Wilcox, S., & Frongillo, E. A. (2015). Comparative effectiveness of plant-based diets for weight loss: A randomized controlled trial of five different diets. *Nutrition, 31*(2), 350–358. https://doi.org/10.1016/j.nut.2014.09.002

U.S. Department of Agriculture. (2020, October 30). *FoodData Central.* fdc.nal.usda.gov. https://fdc.nal.usda.gov/fdc-app.html#/food-details/1100970/nutrients

University of Michigan Health. (2015). *Types of fats.* Uofmhealth.org. https://www.uofmhealth.org/health-library/aa160619

Walder, C. (2020a, April 13). *Healthy zucchini bread steel cut oatmeal.* Walder Wellness. https://www.walderwellness.com/healthy-zucchini-bread-steel-cut-oatmeal/

Walder, C. (2020b, December 29). *Banana chai smoothie with vanilla*. Walder Wellness. https://www.walderwellness.com/banana-chai-smoothie-vanilla/

Webster, K. (2018, April). *Tofu kebabs with zucchini and eggplant*. EatingWell. https://www.eatingwell.com/recipe/264137/tofu-kebabs-with-zucchini-eggplant/

Whitbread, D. (2021, July 28). *Top 10 foods highest in calories to avoid for weight loss*. Myfooddata. https://www.myfooddata.com/articles/high-calorie-foods-to-avoid.php

Wise, J. (2015). Vegetarians have lower risk of colorectal cancers, study finds. *BMJ*, *350*(mar09 10), h1313–h1313. https://doi.org/10.1136/bmj.h1313

Wu, H.-J., & Wu, E. (2012). The role of gut microbiota in immune homeostasis and autoimmunity. *Gut Microbes*, *3*(1), 4–14. https://doi.org/10.4161/gmic.19320

Zheng, D., Liwinski, T., & Elinav, E. (2020). Interaction between microbiota and immunity in health and disease. *Cell Research*, *30*(6), 492–506. https://doi.org/10.1038/s41422-020-0332-7